Natural Relief
for Your
Child's Asthma

Natural Relief
for Your
Child's Asthma

A GUIDE TO CONTROLLING SYMPTOMS & REDUCING YOUR CHILD'S DEPENDENCE ON DRUGS

STEVEN J. BOCK, M.D.,

KENNETH BOCK, M.D.,

AND NANCY PAULINE BRUNING

A LYNN SONBERG BOOK

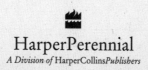

HarperPerennial

A Division of HarperCollinsPublishers

HarperCollins books may be purchased for educational, business, or sales promotional use. For information please write: Special Markets Department, HarperCollins Publishers, Inc., 10 East 53rd Street, New York, NY 10022.

FIRST EDITION

Designed by Christine Weathersbee
Illustrations by North Market Street Graphics

Library of Congress Cataloging-in-Publication Data

Bock, Steven J.
    Natural relief for your child's asthma : a guide to controlling symptoms and reducing your child's dependence on drugs / Steven J. Bock, Kenneth Bock, and Nancy Pauline Bruning.
      p. cm.
    Includes bibliographical references.
    ISBN 0-06-095289-X
    1. Asthma in children—popular works. 2. Asthma in children—Alternative treatment—popular works. I. Bock, Kenneth, 1953– II. Bruning, Nancy Pauline. III. Title.
RJ436.A68B63 1999
618.92'238—dc21   98-43771

99 00 01 02 03 ❖/RRD 10 9 8 7 6 5 4 3 2 1

IMPORTANT NOTE:

This book is not intended to take the place of medical advice from a trained medical professional. We recommend that all readers interested in natural approaches to asthma care seek the guidance of a qualified health professional before implementing any of the approaches to health suggested in this book. Since research about natural and medical approaches to treating asthma is ongoing and subject to conflicting interpretations, there is no guarantee that what we know about this complex subject won't change with time. Neither the publisher, the producer, nor the authors take any responsibility for any treatment, action, or application of medicine or preparation by any person reading or following the information in this book. The names of parents and their patients have been changed.

CONTENTS

ACKNOWLEDGMENTS

The authors wish to thank:
Peter A. Kaplan, Psy.D., clinical psychologist and director
of the mind-body department of our progressive medicine centers,
and Vicki Koenig, M.S., R.D., certified dietitian and nutritionist, for
their contribution to the care of our patients as well as to the book.

Drs. Steven and Kenneth Bock wish to thank:
Our parents, Fred and Nora; our wives, Kerri and Marian; and our
children, Aaron, Anna, Rebecca, Isabelle, Alicia, and Jordan for
their support and patience during the writing of this book, and
our patients, who teach us so much and without
whom this book could not have been written.

Nancy Pauline Bruning would like to acknowledge
her mother, Anna, and J.B.

INTRODUCTION

If you are the parent of a child with asthma, you know what it is like to watch someone you love be at constant risk of having to fight for air: her breath is labored, she coughs constantly and perhaps wheezes, she perspires profusely, her tiny chest and neck are "sucked in" with each precious breath. You may live in constant anxiety because such episodes are unpredictable. When will the next episode occur? How severe will it be? Will it happen at school, while she's playing or doing her homework, or while she's sleeping peacefully? Will she be able to catch her breath? Will she die? Will she be like this the rest of her life?

Such uncertainty and potentially serious consequences mean your whole family can get caught in a spiral of symptoms, panic, anxiety, medication, doctor and emergency-room visits, lost sleep, worry, and isolation. In our practice we have seen how stressed and desperate a parent can get—you'll do *anything* to help your child breathe again. As a result, parents have felt they had no alternative but to give their child conventional antiasthma medications.

And what powerful drugs they are! During the fifteen years we have been treating children with asthma, there have been remarkable advances made in the medical treatment of asthma. Recently a whole new class of drugs has been introduced, and researchers are developing better ways of administering them. That's why today most children with asthma take one or more prescription or over-the-counter medications that aim to prevent or relieve asthma flare-ups. While these medications can be life-saving and life enhancing for many children, the parents of our young patients have been troubled by the idea of giving their children drugs on a regular basis. The fact that you are reading this book shows that you have joined their ranks. You are right to be concerned. Although drugs can be useful and even lifesaving, they do have their downside.

It's been widely acknowledged that these drugs can have immediate side effects such as mood swings, restlessness, and irregular heartbeat; these risks have been considered to be relatively minor and reversible and therefore generally thought to be worth the potential benefit. However, recent scientific studies have revealed that conventional drugs can cause serious long-term effects, including bone loss, cataracts, and glaucoma. And contrary to popular belief, most children do not completely "grow out of" asthma—despite conventional treatment, their asthma grows worse, or returns after a brief hiatus, setting children on a path of lifelong dependency on medical care and medication, of worrying that another crisis may be just around the corner. What parent wouldn't be distressed at such a prospect?

As progressive physicians we long ago started asking: if these drugs are the answer, why is the rate and severity of asthma increasing? The fact is, the number of people suffering from asthma has *doubled* since the early 1980s. The rate of emergency room visits and hospitalizations has gone up, and children in such dire circumstances are requiring more powerful treatments. Asthma now affects 17.3 million Americans—at least five million of them are children. Today, it's not unusual to see children toting inhalers and peak flow meters to school. Even with medication, ten million school days are lost annually. And parents lose one billion dollars a year staying home from work to care for their asthmatic children. What's wrong with this picture?

It is our belief that asthma rates continue to soar because of our increasingly toxic environment. Our children are assaulted from every direction with indoor and outdoor air pollution, poor food, and stress. This accumulating toxicity affects all their systems, making them more vulnerable to diseases, such as asthma, to which they have a genetic predisposition. Ironically, asthma drugs themselves add to the toxic burden, causing not only the previously mentioned side effects, but also worsening the underlying imbalance that leads to asthma in the first place. Furthermore, conventional therapies, although usually effective in the short term, treat symptoms by suppressing them; they do nothing to treat the underlying condition. Ultimately, they create a dependency on medication, physicians, and hospitals that takes a terrible emotional and financial toll.

This is clearly not good news. However, there *is* a way that you and your child can lessen your child's dependence on medication, improve her general health, and gain a greater sense of control over asthma. That way is to follow our Natural Asthma Control Program, a program we have developed from years of study, observation, and experience, that integrates natural medical approaches and conventional medical care.

As board-certified physicians and leaders in progressive medicine, we have extensive training and experience in both conventional and alternative medicine. We have seen firsthand the advantages and limitations of each form of medicine and have found that using a multidimensional approach to be superior to either one alone. We have been developing and refining this natural asthma control program for our collective thirty years of clinical experience. Working with our staff, which includes a certified dietitian-nutritionist and a clinical psychologist, at our two health centers in upstate New York, we have been helping parents incorporate allergy control, nutrition, herbs, homeopathy, and mind-body therapies with appropriate conventional treatment. Through using this progressive, integrated approach, we have helped hundreds of parents and children control asthma naturally and reduce their use of asthma medication. On our program, children who were on the road to a lifetime of drug dependency now have fewer episodes of asthma symptoms, and episodes are milder and of shorter duration. In some cases they only use an inhaler for those rare times when symptoms flare; some children are completely free of medication. What's more, our young patients are in better physical and emotional health and have assumed greater responsibility and control, thus diminishing the sense of powerlessness, helplessness, and panic that so often otherwise characterizes living with a serious chronic illness. Thanks to natural therapies, they live fuller, more normal, happy, productive lives—and so do their entire families.

But we can only educate and treat a limited number of patients. That's why we have teamed up with a veteran writer who has authored or coauthored twenty books, most of them on health topics. Together we have developed a book that is easy to read, simple to follow, and provides a step-by-step program that shows how you and your children can gradually lessen your reliance on drugs and "crisis" care. This is the first book that deals exclusively with children suffering from asthma and provides a comprehensive program that you can safely and confidently follow on your own, in your own home. We not only teach you about the true nature and causes of asthmatic episodes, we show you how you can safely and confidently introduce gentle, effective, natural therapies into your daily routine and integrate them with regular conventional medical care.

The goal of our program is to relieve and prevent symptoms of asthma and reduce reliance on prescription drugs. To accomplish this, we give you a working knowledge of asthma, its treatment, and the most effective natural approaches used to control the condition. Throughout, we offer you the psychological and practical support they need to confidently and safely make the lifestyle and attitude changes that are needed to control your child's asthma naturally.

In the first chapter we supply basic information about asthma. This includes a description of asthma, its symptoms and the underlying mechanism that causes them, and how environmental and emotional toxic overload makes some children more prone to asthma than others. In the next chapter we discuss the accomplishments and limitations of conventional treatment, and in the third chapter we recommend certain preliminary steps to help you prepare to integrate natural therapies in your child's overall treatment plan. Following that, we devote a chapter explaining how to use this book to create an individualized treatment and prevention program uniquely suited to your child and your family.

The next six chapters are devoted to describing the safest, most effective, and most readily available natural therapies used to treat and prevent asthma, and explain how you can integrate them into your child's life along with current medical therapy. These chapters show you: how to detoxify your child's environment and avoid common triggers such as pollen, dust mites, and mold; how foods can either help heal your child's asthma or harm and actually trigger episodes directly or indirectly; the role of nutritional supplements—how, for example, vitamins C, E, and beta-carotene, essential fatty acids, and flavonoids can reduce inflammation and protect cells from damage, decreasing asthma episodes and minimizing the harmful side effects of antiasthma drugs; the most effective herbs and other plant-based remedies used to reduce the risk of asthma flare-ups, and as the first line of treatment should symptoms appear, as well as a summary of what homeopathy has to offer as a cure and for symptom relief; how to deal with toxic stressful emotions that are part of living with asthma, as either cause or effect; and mind-body medicines to melt away stress and imagine away symptoms.

The final chapter consists of the stories of three of our patients, as told by their parents, who used natural therapies successfully. We hope that these true life stories will inspire you and motivate you to embark on your own Natural Asthma Control Program.

In the last section we have gathered a wealth of hard-to-find resources for parents and their children: a glossary of terms, reference notes, a suggested reading list, plus where to look for more information, support, products, practitioners, and services.

Natural Relief for Your Child's Asthma is the first book written for parents who, with professional medical guidance, want to reduce—and, possibly, eventually replace—conventional medical treatment by using natural, remedies. This book will help you understand what is happening with your child and show you how you can safely use alternative therapies to improve the quality of life for your asthmatic child and for the whole family. As a caring parent, you need to know that your precious child can live a more normal, active, happy life— without selling short his or her future. *Natural Relief for Your Child's Asthma* will give you this gift.

IMPORTANT NOTE:

In this book, safety and the welfare of the child always comes first. Because of the nature of the ailment, we will give precautions wherever necessary to ensure the well-being of the child. *Do not abandon ongoing medical treatment.* Complementary therapies are just that—they complement conventional care but are not intended to replace it or the advice and information you receive from your medical and health-care professionals. Because asthma can disable and even kill, we recognize that conventional treatment may be necessary during a severe flare-up, and we provide clear warning signs when medication or professional attention is necessary.

ONE   UNDERSTANDING ASTHMA

In our experience, the better a parent and child understand asthma and its causes, the better able they are to use our Natural Asthma Control Program to prevent and alleviate symptoms and reduce dependency on medications. Education and understanding are so important to success that, in a sense, you are already beginning the program just by reading this chapter.

We first explain the most current understanding of the causes of asthma and what happens during a flare-up. We tell you who gets asthma and provide you with a basic understanding of how your child's lungs and immune system differ from that of a child without asthma. We then explain the theory behind what we believe to be the underlying cause of asthma—toxic overload. With this basic foundation of knowledge, you will be better able to communicate with your child's doctor and together devise a treatment plan. You will better understand the following chapter on how medications work. And you will understand the rationale behind each action step in the program and how it affects the whole picture.

Once you have a basic understanding of asthma, talk to your child about asthma and explain, in terms that he can understand, what asthma is. Then talk to him about the changes you'll be making in order to better control the condition so he can live a more normal life.

ASTHMA BASICS

Asthma is a lung disorder that results in recurrent episodes of breathing difficulty. Asthma is not a new illness: Over two thousand years ago the Greeks knew of this condition and coined the word *asthma* from a Greek word that means "to pant." Indeed, shortness of breath is one of the primary symptoms of this respiratory disorder, along with coughing, wheezing, and a tight feeling in the chest.

Although asthma is generally characterized by these telltale symptoms, the actual symptoms and their severity vary from person to person. And they vary within any individual, becoming worse during an asthma episode or flare-up. (We dislike the word "attack," a frightening term which can make people of all ages feel like helpless victims.) Asthma flare-ups may last a few minutes or for days at a time and can even be life threatening. In some children, asthma is mild and only bothers them some of the time. For others, each day is a struggle to breathe. Even in mild cases, it is life disrupting.

As one adult who had asthma as a child recalls, "Fear wasn't so much the issue—I always felt I could get the air—I just had to work very hard to get it. You need to think about and focus on something that should be effortless and automatic. You learn to limit your activity. You simply sit and concentrate on breathing. It's as if nothing exists in the world but you and your breath."

If your child has asthma, you may have asthma yourself and know all too well what a flare-up feels like. It's not like the out-of-breath feeling you get from running too fast; in that case, your lungs are working and with time you do catch your breath. Rather, children and adults describe an asthma episode as "trying to breathe through a narrow straw," or "putting a plastic bag over my head and cutting off my breathing." If you don't have asthma, it's hard to imagine what it feels like physically and emotionally to have difficulty breathing. One way to experience what a bad episode feels like is to take a deep breath and then try to take another breath without letting the first breath out.

Long misunderstood and misdiagnosed, today we know much more about asthma, and that knowledge tells us that asthma is much more complex than originally thought to be. Simply put, asthma is a chronic condition of the lungs that causes the airways to become narrow, resulting in less space for the air to flow in and out. The cause seems to be a combination of genetic predisposition and environmental factors that begin to affect a child as early as infancy—and possibly in the womb.

In a person with asthma, the lungs are unusually sensitive to certain substances called *triggers*. The lungs overreact and are said to be "twitchy"—much like a nervous, sensitive person who jumps at the slightest noise. This overreaction leads to *inflammation*, which is the underlying mechanism of asthma.

Almost anything can trigger asthma, but each child has his own set of triggers. Common triggers include pollens, pet dander, smoke and air

SIGNS AND SYMPTOMS OF ASTHMA

These are the most common symptoms of asthma; they worsen during an episode or flare-up. Although wheezing is usually thought of as characteristic of asthma, not all children with asthma wheeze; and not all have trouble breathing, either. Coughing may be the main or only symptom, especially if it occurs after exercise or during the night. This is sometimes referred to as "cough-variant asthma."

- cough that lasts for more than a week
- recurrent shortness of breath
- recurrent wheezing
- recurrent feeling of tightness in the chest

pollution, gases, fumes, perfumes, colds and flu, cold air, exercise, and foods. Although there is a psychological component to asthma, the condition is not provoked primarily by emotional or psychological stress.

Who Gets Asthma?

Current estimates are that over one hundred million people suffer from this condition worldwide. Asthma affects more than seventeen million Americans; approximately one-third of them—five million—are under the age of sixteen, making it the nation's single leading cause of chronic illness in children. Incredibly, today nearly one out of every fourteen American children aged five to fourteen has asthma. In certain areas, especially big cities, the proportion is even higher. For example, in the Bronx, New York, 25 percent of children (one out of four) have the condition.

Genes play a role in whether a child will develop asthma. Scientists have long noticed that the tendency towards asthma runs in families—if a child has one parent with asthma, his chances of developing asthma are one in four, or three to six times the risk of other children. If both his parents have asthma, his odds are one in two, or ten times the average risk. A child may also inherit *atopy*, which is a tendency to develop the types of allergies that trigger asthma. These include the skin condition known as eczema, hay fever, and food allergies. Recently, several genes have been identified that appear to be related to a child's tendency to develop asthma. So, if your child has asthma, it's because he or she was born with a predisposition for it. However, not every child with this genetic predisposition will go on to actually develop asthma. And not every asthmatic child is born to an allergic or asthmatic family. Environmental and lifestyle factors can clearly play a crucial role in the development of this condition.

Living with a person who smokes boosts the odds that a child will develop asthma. Studies show that up to 25 percent of children with asthma have a parent who smokes, and children who live with mothers who smoke double the risk of developing asthma. Other factors that increase the risk of a child developing asthma are having a severe viral infection during infancy and being born premature, both of which compromise the lungs, leaving them more sensitive and "twitchy." Fifty to 70 percent of children with asthma experience their first episode by the time they are three years old.

The incidence of asthma has been increasing all over the world among all age groups, particularly in industrialized areas. According to the American Medical Association, the asthma rate in the United States nearly tripled from 1980 to 1994 among those aged five to twenty-four. It is now the most prevalent chronic disorder affecting children between birth and seventeen years of age. In spite of medical advances in the treatment of asthma, the severity of asthma has increased as well. Five times as many children are hospitalized for asthma symptoms than twenty years ago, and they are requiring more dramatic and powerful medical treatment.

The Impact of Asthma

Childhood asthma causes more hospital admissions, more visits to hospital emergency rooms, and more school absences than any other chronic childhood disease. The medical cost of treating asthma in American children under eighteen years of age is nearly $2 billion a year. Overall, asthma costs $6.2 billion each year in treatment and days lost from work—about 1 percent of the total spent on all illnesses in the United States.

Asthma can even kill if it is not brought under control. Today, asthma kills five thousand Americans every year—nearly twice the rate in 1979. And many of them are children.

Just as important, asthma can severely disrupt the living patterns of entire families, preventing children from living normal, happy, active lives and interfering with their full physical, social, mental, and emotional development. Even if we just look at hospital admissions alone, an asthmatic's life is not a happy one. According to the American Medical Association, asthmatic children under the age of fifteen underwent 159,000 hospitalizations in 1994, with an average stay of 3.4 days. Clearly, this is no life for a tender young child to be living.

DO CHILDREN OUTGROW ASTHMA?

On the upside, as they get older, some children find that their symptoms lessen. A number of factors are responsible for this. Their lungs become more mature and better able to resist allergic inflammation. Their breathing tubes grow larger and less narrow. As their immune systems mature, they become less allergic. And finally, the viruses that trigger asthma are less harmful to older children and adults. By the time they are teenagers, some children seem to be completely free of asthma. In other cases, however, asthma that has become quiescent may become reactivated. This is because the tendency for twitchy, overreactive airways remains throughout life. As a result, individuals may have isolated episodes now and then when they are exposed to a particularly potent trigger or group of triggers.

A CLOSER LOOK AT ASTHMA

Asthma involves the respiratory system and the immune system. By understanding how these two systems normally work in harmony and then how in asthma these systems can go awry, you'll have a clearer picture of why symptoms occur, why your child may suffer certain indirect effects such as lack of energy and hampered growth, and how treatment works.

In a child with normal lungs and respiratory system, air flows freely in and out through airways that branch smaller and smaller, like an upside-down tree.

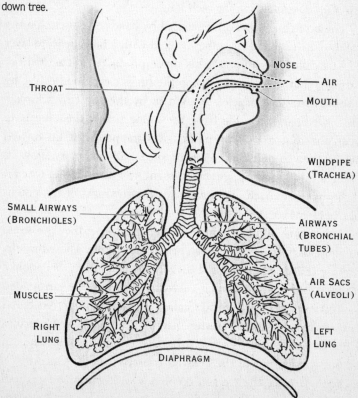

NOSE

THROAT

AIR

MOUTH

WINDPIPE
(TRACHEA)

SMALL AIRWAYS
(BRONCHIOLES)

AIRWAYS
(BRONCHIAL
TUBES)

AIR SACS
(ALVEOLI)

MUSCLES

RIGHT
LUNG

LEFT
LUNG

DIAPHRAGM

THE NORMAL RESPIRATORY SYSTEM

Unless you are asthmatic yourself and are experiencing symptoms as you read this, you are utterly unaware of your breath. Yet without the steady inhale and exhale of this basic life function, you would die. During each inhale-exhale cycle, a miracle of nature happens. As you take in the air through your nose or mouth, it is "conditioned"— warmed and humidified to prepare it for the rest of its journey. It then passes through your throat and *trachea* (windpipe) and enters the lungs through a system of air passages called the *bronchial tubes*. The largest tubes are the two *bronchi* (singular, *bronchus*), one for each lung.

The bronchial tubes are encircled by bands of muscles on the outside. The inside of the tubes is lined with a thin, delicate layer of tissue called the *mucosa*. This tissue produces mucus, a sticky substance that is designed to keep the lungs clean and healthy by trapping irritating particles brought in by the air. Tiny whiplike hairs called *cilia* protrude from the lining tissue; their job is to sweep the mucus and the particulates trapped in it up toward your trachea so you can cough or sneeze it out, or swallow it. (Though this is an unappetizing thought, rest assured that when it reaches your stomach, digestive acids destroy most of the potential troublemakers.)

The bronchial tubes branch smaller the deeper they penetrate the lungs, like the branches of an upside-down tree. These tiny airways are called *bronchioles* and they finally end in tiny, balloonlike air sacs called *alveoli* (singular, *alveolus*). The sacs are surrounded by a network of blood vessels called capillaries. Your red blood cells pass through the capillaries, marching in single file. Molecules of life-giving oxygen pass from the alveoli into the bloodstream and are transported to the cells all over your body. Once it has reached the cells, the oxygen combines with carbohydrates and fats to release their energy. This energy is needed by the cells for many processes and is the basis of life.

Meanwhile, the cells produce carbon dioxide as a waste product and dump molecules of this gas into the blood. Transported by the circulatory system to the lungs, the molecules of carbon dioxide enter the alveoli, the bronchioles, and then the bronchi. Your body rids itself of carbon dioxide with each exhale.

To breathe, you need to use your chest muscles. During the inhale, your rib muscles and diaphragm contract; this increases the volume of your chest cavity, which decreases the air pressure in the chest. Oxygen rushes into the alveoli, forcing them to expand like tiny balloons. During the exhale, your rib muscles and diaphragm relax, shrinking the volume of your chest cavity. This increases the air pressure in your chest, compressing the alveoli and forcing the carbon dioxide out.

WHAT HAPPENS DURING AN ASTHMA FLARE-UP?

In asthma, the respiratory system and immune system overreact to substances such as pollen, dust, and infection. These triggers stimulate an all-out defense in which *inflammation* plays a central and continuing role. Inflammation leads to *mucus formation* and *bronchial constriction*, two other mechanisms designed to protect us. Scientists used to believe that bronchoconstriction caused asthma symptoms and inflammation. We now know that it's the other way around: inflammation occurs first. Asthma, it seems, is basically an inflammatory disease. We also have come to think of asthma as both *chronic* and *episodic*. By chronic we mean the tendency for your child's airways to be inflamed is always there; by episodic we mean that every now and then the inflamed lungs flare up into a distinct asthma episode. If your child's body is constantly exposed to triggers, her body is constantly reactive—actually overreactive; her lungs are inflamed because of the constant barrage of inflammatory chemicals. This environment of inflammation is like a smoldering fire. Although there may be no symptoms, or only mild symptoms, the lungs remain on red alert, teetering on the brink of a flare-up. This sets the stage for a trigger to come along and fan the flames like a gust of wind, turning the smoldering fire into a big flare-up with obvious symptoms of coughing, wheezing, and shortness of breath.

In the normally functioning lung, inflammation, mucus production, and bronchoconstriction exist in order to protect us from harm. In an asthmatic child the normal defense mechanisms are simply too sensitive and excitable, and their activity is out of proportion to the actual danger. Here's how these three mechanisms work in concert to cause the airways to become irritated and narrower from the inside and the outside, leading to coughing, wheezing, and trouble breathing.

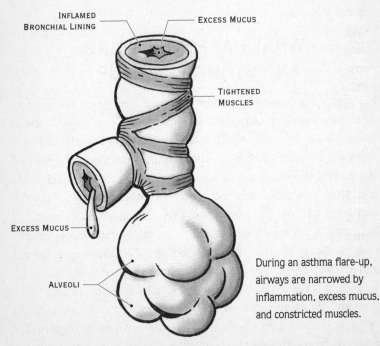

INFLAMED BRONCHIAL LINING

EXCESS MUCUS

TIGHTENED MUSCLES

EXCESS MUCUS

ALVEOLI

During an asthma flare-up, airways are narrowed by inflammation, excess mucus, and constricted muscles.

Inflammation

The airways of children with asthma are usually sensitive, and they also contain more inflammatory cells than other children's. Once stimulated, the cells signal the body to send more inflammatory cells from the immune system to flood the area. The extra cells and extra fluid they produce cause redness, heat, and swelling, making the airway narrower. At this point, air can still pass through the tubes, and there may be no symptoms or just mild symptoms such as a cough, some chest tightness, or less energy than usual.

Mucus Production

Next, the mucus membrane lining the inside of the tubes forms extra mucus to protect the irritated tissue. Unfortunately, the extra mucus also hampers the ability of the lungs to absorb oxygen and expel carbon dioxide and, along with the immune cells and injured cells, creates a formidable amount of debris that narrows the passageways further. This excess mucus is a key symptom, and, using a stethoscope, you or your child's doctor can hear the mucus "rattle around" the bronchial tubes.

Muscle Constriction

Meanwhile, the nerves in the area also become irritated from the onslaught of inflammatory cells, and in response the muscles surrounding the bronchial tubes go into spasm. As they contract and squeeze, the airways narrow even more. This is also called *bronchospasm* or *bronchoconstriction*. Your child's fragile alveoli begin to strangle from the pressure and she coughs and gasps for air. Bronchoconstriction is also caused by allergies such as pollen and exposure to irritating substances such as paint fumes.

KEY COMPONENTS OF INFLAMMATION

Once stimulated by an invader, specialized cells in the body unleash a barrage of powerful chemicals. Here are the key players:

Macrophage: The first cell to discover an invader and alert helper T-cells.

Helper T-cell: The immune cell that stimulates the B-cells to produce antibodies.

Antibodies: Also called immunoglobulins, these are the initial chemicals released by immune cells called B-cells that initiate the inflammatory response.

Immunoglobulin E (IgE): An antibody secreted during response to an allergen.

Cytokines: The name given to a group of inflammatory chemicals released by immune cells, triggered by antibodies.

Prostaglandins: Inflammatory chemicals that cause the initial stage of inflammation.

Histamine: An inflammatory chemical that attracts additional immune cells to the site; histamine also irritates the nerves that control the muscles surrounding the airways, causing them to constrict, and stimulates the secretion of mucus.

Leukotrienes: Chemicals that appear to constrict the muscles encircling the airways and increase mucus production. (Leukotriene is the basis of a new medical treatment for asthma.)

Neutrophils: Immune cells that isolate and ingest bacteria.

Mast cells: Immune cells that release inflammatory chemicals including histamine and leukotrienes.

Suppressor T-cells: T-cells that "turn off" B-cells and end the inflammatory process.

Inflammation, Allergy, and Asthma

Understanding inflammation is the key to understanding asthma and its treatment. Under normal circumstances, inflammation is also one of the body's most potent mechanisms for protecting the lungs from harmful substances such as viruses and irritating fumes. It also appears to be the link between allergies and asthma.

Inflammation is part of the immune response. It occurs after a harmful substance enters the respiratory system and evades the initial excretory defense mechanism of the mucus and cilia, when the specialized cells of the immune system swing into action. Immune cells along your respiratory tract secrete *antibodies*, which set in motion a cascade of events. When inflammation occurs in the lungs, it can narrow the airways, causing symptoms of asthma. A variety of cells speed to the area and secrete various chemicals (see "Key Components of Inflammation" on page 12). Some of these chemicals cause the area to flood with fluid, causing swelling. Some stimulate the production of mucus, which plugs the airways. Still others cause the bronchioles to constrict.

Eighty percent of people with asthma also have allergies, and it appears that allergies and allergic-like reactions can trigger asthma. As with asthma itself, an allergic reaction represents the body's defense system gone awry. An allergy is a type of reaction that develops gradually in a child who has inherited the tendency to be allergic. We don't yet understand exactly why, but with repeated exposure, the body becomes "sensitized" to a harmless substance, such as pollen, and reacts as if it were a harmful one.

Substances that provoke allergic reactions are called *allergens*. As with any invader perceived as harmful, the immune system develops an antibody in response to the allergen. Children with allergies seem to produce an overabundance of an antibody called immunoglobulin E (IgE). The IgE antibody to the allergen attaches to receptors on mast cells. Whenever the mast cells are again exposed to the allergen, the allergen molecule links up two adjacent antibodies attached to the same mast cell. This allergen-antibody pairing, or "complex," signals the mast cells to churn out inflammatory chemicals such as prostaglandins, histamine, and leukotrienes, which can narrow the airways.

It may also be that the chemicals released during an infection or allergic reaction leave the lungs inflamed and primed so that the next trigger that comes along can set them off and lead to wheezing and breathlessness.

Airborne allergens that trigger asthma must be too small to be filtered out by the cilia and mucosa, and they must be present in large enough quantities and for a long enough time to cause sensitization. Once sensitization has occurred, however, it takes only a brief exposure to a very small amount to provoke an allergic reaction and lead to an asthma flare-up. Although hay fever–type allergies from pollens, dust, and mold are prime asthma triggers, allergens do not necessarily need to affect the respiratory system to cause asthma. Allergic reactions to foods and medications can cause inflammatory swelling throughout the entire body, including the airways, causing bronchoconstriction and wheezing.

Allergy is not the same as *irritation*, which does not involve IgE but does cause inflammation and bronchoconstriction. People with twitchy, hypersensitive lungs are prone to irritation, so irritation can be a trigger in people who are not allergic in the classic sense.

WHY IT'S IMPORTANT
TO CONTROL ASTHMA

Each child has her own unique patterns of asthma lulls, mild symptoms, and serious flare-ups. With proper treatment, these patterns can even out so there are fewer dramatic ups and downs.

Your child may be totally symptom free between episodes, or the underlying inflammation may cause mild or moderate symptoms such as a nagging or intermittent cough or chest tightness. Flare-ups may last less than an hour or drag on for weeks; they may be serious enough to interrupt your child's activities and require that she take a rest. She may need to take medicine in order to breathe normally again. Sometimes a flare-up is so serious that the decreased oxygen she is getting is life threatening, and she may need to be taken to the emergency room of the hospital for treatment. Fortunately, it is rare for a fatal episode to come on suddenly; usually symptoms get worse over a period of hours or days, giving plenty of warning time to get the proper treatment, provided you know what to look for.

Another reason it's important to control asthma is to avoid the upper respiratory infections that are a common complication of asthma in children. Viral infections often trigger or worsen asthma symptoms, but it also works the other way around. During a prolonged asthma episode, mucus becomes trapped in the airways, and this becomes a breeding site for bacteria, which can cause secondary infection such as strep throat.

Though distressing, these are only the most obvious and immediate reasons to control asthma. Other effects are more subtle or delayed. Even when asthma is mild, your child may not be getting the oxygen she needs. She has to work extra hard to get oxygen into her lungs and into her system. This struggle, even when it takes place on a subtle level, can contribute to the fatigue that so often plagues children with asthma. The struggle for air pursues them even in their sleep, and often an asthmatic child will awaken in the middle of the night because she is unable to breathe. Shortchanged of the vital oxygen needed to convert food into energy so that organs can grow, she may be smaller than average. In some children, the lungs are less able to repair themselves after each asthmatic episode, particularly if they are exposed to cigarette smoke or harmful levels of air pollution. When the tissue becomes severely damaged, it repairs itself by forming new tissue. But this tissue is like scar tissue—harder and thicker than the original—and it is permanent. In addition, her immune system may become less and less able to tolerate a greater variety of allergens and other triggers.

So, asthma is not simply a question of "shortness of breath." It can affect your child's health and well-being in many ways for many years—perhaps her whole life. And fixing asthma isn't a matter of giving your child medication that temporarily eases breathing. That's why we urge you and our patients to incorporate natural treatments into any asthma control program. By adding natural medicines we can get to the root of asthma and provide consistent, long-term relief and prevention of asthma symptoms and related conditions.

WHY THE INCREASE?: TOXIC OVERLOAD

While millions of children suffer from asthma and thousands more are diagnosed each year, the medical community continues to debate why some children's immune systems go haywire, inflaming airways, constricting breathing tubes, and interfering with their ability to breathe. No one is completely sure why asthma is increasing so dramatically. However, many scientists, ourselves included, believe that the increasing level of toxins in our environment plays a major role. As Stephen C. Redd, of the U.S. Centers for Disease Control and Prevention, said: "The genetic makeup of the population couldn't have changed enough to see the increases that are being seen in many developed countries. So there's got to be some kind of environmental exposure."

The increase in environmental toxins could also help explain the disparity in the incidence of asthma between low- and high-income neighborhoods. Dr. Andrew Aligne, of Rochester General Hospital and University of Rochester in Rochester, New York, has found that children living in the city have a higher rate than is average for children generally, regardless of race or income level. Again, this points to something in the children's environment, something that has changed enough over the last twenty years to have doubled the incidence of asthma.

More Toxins Everywhere

We believe that asthma isn't caused by a change in any one thing, but that it is multifactorial. It's fairly typical for a child today to live in a house that is heavily insulated; it contains new wall-to-wall carpeting and has just been repainted. She rides to school in a diesel bus and occasionally breathes in a big gulp of fumes. At school, she sits next to a rabbit in homeroom. She doesn't like her vegetables and doesn't take vitamins, and she drinks large quantities of soft drinks. Although anyone would consider her to be "well off," her life is full of asthma triggers. Her poor immune system is so overloaded her body can't help but respond with chronic inflammation, coughing, wheezing, and constricted airways in a last-ditch attempt to deal with the poisons.

In fact, so many factors have changed in recent decades that it would be quite surprising if we weren't seeing more asthma in our patients: not only is the air and water more polluted but food is less nutritious and contains synthetic chemicals, and changes in the way society and families function are creating an unprecedented stress on vulnerable children. In our practice of natural medicine, we consider allergies and asthma to be part of a continuum of increased hypersensitivity to our increasingly hostile, toxic environment. Toxic overload may be partially responsible for the astounding increase in the rate of childhood cancers—1 percent per year in the last two decades, according to a recent report by the National Cancer Institute.

Broadly speaking, toxins are anything that harms or "poisons" the body, and a variety of factors act like toxins in the body. Toxins can be substances that enter the body from the outside through air, water, and food. Or they can be chemicals the body produces itself. For example, toxins are formed when the body produces free radicals.

Free Radicals and Inflammation

Free radicals cause destruction in the body. These highly reactive charged particles are missing an electron. They are quite unstable and steal electrons from neighboring molecules, turning them into more free radicals in the process. The new crop of free radicals in turn steal electrons from their neighbors, and so on, creating a chain reaction that ultimately destroys tissue, such as lung tissue, by oxidizing it. Free radicals create inflammation, and inflammation in turn creates free radicals in an endless cycle of destruction.

We're exposed to free radicals from indoor and outdoor air pollution, pollutants in our food and water, alcohol, drugs, cigarette smoke, and radiation. Free radicals form when fats and other substances combine with oxygen in the body. Our bodies also produce them during normal metabolism; for example, white blood cells produce free radicals to fight invaders such as viruses and bacteria. Thus, free radicals are needed for survival; however, they are dangerous when there are too many of them and they overload our system. Free radicals can attack any component of the cell—including the genetic material in the nucleus, cell walls, and other components, and particularly those parts that contain polyunsaturated fatty acids (PUFAs). When unchecked, free radicals generate more free radicals, and this chain reaction creates free radical overload. Cells may die, malfunction, or become cancerous; tissues and organs may be damaged. Your immune system, whose job it is to clean up and remove damaged cells, is overburdened. The organs of the immune system may themselves be damaged by free radicals. Free radical damage, also called oxidation, is what causes metal to rust, rubber to turn brittle, butter to turn rancid, and paintings to deteriorate. In the human body it has been associated with immune problems and many diseases and conditions including premature aging and death, cardiovascular disease, many types of cancer, diabetes, cataracts and other degenerative eye problems, arthritis, and possibly osteoporosis. Free radicals are involved in the inflammation that is the underlying cause of asthma but, as you will see in later chapters of this book, natural therapies help keep free radicals under control.

Chemical Pollutants

One group of toxins, synthetic chemicals, is particularly troubling. Every day people breathe in these by-products of increasing industrialization and development—thousands of them, including auto exhaust, industrial wastes, insecticides, weed killers, household cleaners, and runoff from streets and farms that contaminates drinking water. We eat them and drink them as food preservatives and "enhancers." While in many ways they have improved our lives, such toxic chemicals are growing steadily in amount and number, and they are being introduced faster than humans can adapt to their presence. In many cases, they are not necessary, and nontoxic substitutes exist or could be developed.

"Everyone on the planet is carrying at least two hundred and fifty measurable chemicals in his or her body that were not part of human chemistry before the 1920s," says Pete Meyers, coauthor of the book *Our Stolen Future*. An estimated seventy-five thousand new synthetic chemicals have been introduced in the last half century, and the volume produced in the United States has increased a thousandfold over the last sixty years, according to an article in the *Amicus Journal*. The article goes on to say that in the United States, "[ninety] percent of new industrial and commercial chemicals are approved for production or commercial use without any mandatory health-testing data." In 1997 the Environmental Defense Fund published a report stating that nearly 75 percent of the most widely used chemicals have not undergone even the most basic toxicity testing. If a chemical is tested for toxicity, it is often tested for its cancer-causing ability, and for nothing else. Cancer is a discrete, relatively easily identifiable effect, but there are other possible health effects, such as asthma, neurological damage, and hormone disruption, that are more subtle. These effects often occur at much lower doses than are being tested and accepted as safe. Furthermore, no one knows the effects of low doses of chemicals over the long term, and no one knows precisely what happens when this jumble of chemicals interacts.

Outdoor Air Pollution

Components of smog and air pollution such as ozone, sulfur dioxide, and nitrogen oxide irritate the airways, increase their sensitivity to other substances, cause bronchoconstriction, and increase mucus production. According to the Natural Resources Defense Council, in 1995 almost eighteen million children under the age of ten lived in areas where the air quality did not meet federal standards. The American Lung Association has found that hospital admissions for asthma rise 20 to 30 percent when air pollution worsens. And recent research by Michael Burr of the Center for Applied Public Health Medicine in Cardiff, Wales, indicates asthma is increasing in areas where industrial pollution has improved but auto traffic has worsened. His studies show that industrial pollution with sulfur dioxide and smoke doesn't cause asthma directly but can worsen it, and that diesel exhaust fumes and ozone increase the effects of inhaled allergens.

Air pollution may weaken the general health of the lungs, leaving them more susceptible to asthma. Several studies have shown that the ozone in smog, even in concentrations that are within EPA standards, increases sensitivity to pollens by 200 to 300 percent.

Particulates—as opposed to gaseous fumes—are gaining more attention as respiratory toxins and asthma provokers. The Natural Resources Defense Council estimated in 1996 that nationwide, fine particles from coal-fired plants and gas- and diesel-powered vehicles cause more than fifty-six thousand deaths each year. The people most at risk are those with respiratory illnesses such as asthma. A 1998 study conducted in Canada found that asthmatic children are more susceptible to the effects of particulates than are nonasthmatic children, and at levels far below the current U.S. standard. The smaller the particulates, the deeper they can penetrate into the lungs, where they become embedded and difficult for the immune system to remove, no matter how hard it bombards the lung with inflammatory chemicals. Unfortunately, the EPA regulates "large" particles of air pollution, but not "small" particles.

Indoor Air Pollution

According to the Environmental Protection Agency, today most Americans spend 90 percent of their time indoors, in buildings and in cars. That's a far cry from the "old days" when people often walked from place to place instead of taking cars everywhere, and children played outdoors instead of being glued to the TV, VCR, and video games. Spending more time indoors may seem like a good idea, considering the air pollution outside. But it is not. Studies indicate that the indoor air we breathe is *even worse* than the outdoor air is today, and far worse than it was a few decades ago. There are several factors at play.

Most modern homes and other buildings have more sources of recognized allergens—such as carpets and the pets that we keep indoors most of the time—than in the past. Instead of wood, wool, and cotton, our furnishings, and the very materials used to build the homes, offices, schools, and stores themselves, are made of synthetic materials. Many of these materials lose molecules into the air—a process called outgassing—and then are inhaled. Soft plastics, such as shower curtains, are notorious outgassers. And today's new carpets contain about twenty different chemicals, many of which outgas. Formaldehyde is one of the more common chemicals that outgas. It binds with certain immune system cells and causes an allergic-type reaction in many people. Formaldehyde is found in countless products, including particle-board furniture, many fabrics, oil-based paints, paper towels, detergents, soft plastics such as shower curtains, and perfumed soaps, to name a few.

These chemicals are trapped and concentrated indoors, because in the interest of saving energy to heat and cool our homes, we have made them airtight. This has created "sick building syndrome," a condition that only began to be taken seriously when thirty employees at an office of the EPA became ill from the new carpet's fumes. Heavily insulated homes also make it easy for other common indoor allergens such as dust mites and mold to accumulate.

The breathing of indoor air, perhaps combined with lack of exercise, affects children in many ways. Dr. Thomas Platts-Mills, of the University of Virginia's Asthma and Allergic Diseases Center, has studied communities where asthma has increased. He says that in every one of these communities, children were spending more time being entertained indoors and less time exercising outdoors.

How Toxic Overload Leads to Asthma

A single trigger rarely sets off an asthma flare-up; the stage must be set long before exposure to a trigger by the cumulative effect of other toxins that have created chronic inflammation. Once the stage has been set, triggers worsen the already existing lung inflammation, bronchoconstriction, or excess mucus production.

When we explain the theory of toxic overload to our patients, we suggest that they imagine their child's body to be a rain barrel, and each toxin is a drop of rain. Her body has built-in mechanisms to handle toxins, but only so many. Like too many raindrops causing the barrel to leak or overflow, too many toxins overload a child's body, and the pressure causes various systems to break down.

Children, with their smaller size and immature immune systems, are particularly vulnerable to toxic overload. Some children who have inherited particularly strong constitutions are better able to handle the load. Others are ill-equipped to deal with this onslaught. Children can become so toxic that their livers may lose the ability to detoxify harmful substances, so the substances keep circulating and causing damage and inflammation. The immune system may be so overloaded that it ceases to function well enough to ward off infections or cancer. Somewhere, the barrel will overflow or leak, and if the lung is where a child's constitutional weakness is, that is where the problem will occur, and the result may be asthma.

Although few would advocate we eradicate all synthetic chemicals, we agree with the public-health and environmental advocates who contend that the current chemical regulatory system is too lenient. As it stands now, most chemicals are considered to be innocent until proven guilty, and the burden of proof that they are harmful rests on those being injured. We need to insist that regulations be tightened and encourage innovative, bright people to come up with less toxic alternatives. Federal authorities such as the Environmental Protection Agency are moving to review environmental regulations in an effort to reverse these troubling trends.

In the meantime, there is much that you and your child can do in your own lives to reduce the toxic burden and achieve greater control over asthma.

TWO UNDERSTANDING THE LIMITS OF <u>CONVENTIONAL MEDICINE</u>

When your child is in the throes of a severe asthma episode, there is no doubt that giving her conventional medicine is your best course of action. However, despite advances in the way conventional medicine treats asthma, even the best of the new drugs have their limitations. No matter how effective the drugs are in alleviating immediate symptoms of an asthma crisis, they do nothing to remedy the underlying condition of inflammation and a dysfunctional immune system. By adding to the toxic burden, they may even worsen asthma over the long run. This is exactly the opposite of natural remedies, which work on the underlying condition and help detoxify and strengthen—rather than further poison and weaken—your child's system.

In this chapter we provide you with a synopsis of the drugs used conventionally: what they are, why and how they are used, and their side effects and limitations. Although the goal is to wean your child away from these medications, we feel it is important for you to understand the rationale behind them, their side effects, and the best way to use them. While on the Natural Asthma Control Program, your child will continue to receive conventional medical treatment as you integrate natural therapies into the overall plan. Although ideally your child will eventually be able to control her asthma without using conventional drugs, not all children will be able to make the complete switch to natural therapies for various reasons. So conventional medication may continue to be part of your overall treatment plan, although to a lesser degree.

Therefore, you must be knowledgeable about asthma medication to make sure your child is making the best use of the drugs available, and to understand how, when, and why to use the most appropriate treatment—be that conventional or natural treatment. Misusing conventional treatment can harm your child, in sometimes surprising ways. Obviously, using more than is necessary is harmful in the long run. But so is using a drug too little or too late; this allows your child's condition to escalate to the point where you need more medication to bring it under control than you would have if you had used appropriate medication earlier on.

Jimmy's mother and father are an excellent example of the effort it may take some parents to make peace with conventional medicine. Jimmy was very sick when we began to treat him, so he needed time to gradually reduce his dependency on conventional drugs. And his parents needed time to get smart and adjust their attitude about using them. Here's how his mother described the experience: "His father and I were practically hippies living in the woods, and we were pretty much anti–prescription drug. But we had to get real and educate ourselves about asthma and the drugs that Jimmy was getting. This was serious—life and death. We had to know the pros and cons, to recognize the side effects. I felt I was at the mercy of the ER people. Jimmy wasn't breathing and I felt so vulnerable, so helpless. Your first notion is to go along and get whatever help your child needs. You surrender. But then, you learn to be more assertive and discriminating. We eventually learned how to decide when natural treatments weren't enough and when conventional treatment was appropriate. You can't be a wimp, but you can't sacrifice your child's well-being to purity of principle, either."

Once you understand the drugs your child is taking and how to use them, we recommend that you talk about them with your child. As a way of introducing this program, explain to your child what the drugs are and what the possible side effects are. Let him know that although conventional medications may be necessary at times, you are going to try to keep their use to a minimum and to start using some other therapies that rarely have side effects.

Two Approaches

There have been many changes taking place in conventional medical treatment for asthma, and more changes are underway. Of the 146 medicines being tested for children in 1977, 15 were for asthma, second in number only to drugs for cancer. The most significant change has been brought about by the recognition that asthma is a chronic condition with acute episodes during which symptoms flare up. There is an underlying inflammation in the lungs that is responsible for the chronic aspect, and the inflammation must be treated continually on a daily basis, whether or not there are discernible symptoms. This is in sharp contrast to the earlier treatment strategy that focused exclusively on dilating (opening up) bronchioles, which constrict during the acute stage. These earlier drugs, called bronchodilators, usually act quickly to relieve shortness of breath and have been used on an "as-needed" basis to rescue a child already in the throes of an episode. In the past, children used bronchodilator medicines continuously and relied on them completely to control their asthma. Unfortunately, studies show that bronchodilators have undesirable immediate side effects and may worsen asthma in the long run (see box, "First Better, Then Worse"). Just as bad, they do not address the underlying mechanism of inflammation.

Today, state-of-the art asthma treatment is two-pronged:

> 1: *Prevention:* To prevent episodes by treating inflam-
> mation, or to prevent the allergic reaction that

leads to inflammation. Medications used to achieve this goal are called *preventer* or controller medicines.

2: *Relief:* To relieve symptoms during an episode by dilating the bronchioles. Medications used to achieve this goal are called *reliever* or rescue medicines.

Both preventer and reliever medicines are taken most commonly by inhaler; they may also be taken as pills or syrups. Inhalers are less likely to cause side effects because they direct the medication to the lungs, and much less reaches the rest of the body directly. We certainly applaud the shift in emphasis toward preventing asthma flare-ups by treating the underlying inflammation. However, anti-inflammatory drugs have their problems, too, as you will see. This is why even among conventional physicians, the daily use of anti-inflammatories in children with mild or moderate asthma is controversial, and why we prefer natural methods such as herbs and nutritional supplements to reduce inflammation.

FIRST BETTER, THEN WORSE

Regular use of bronchodilators called beta-agonists has actually been found to cause asthma control to deteriorate, according to a 1990 New Zealand study. Overall, 30 percent of patients who used bronchodilators were better during treatment, compared with 70 percent of those using a placebo (dummy) medication. Recent research also shows that these medications increase bronchial hypersensitivity, especially if given over a long period of time or in large doses.

Preventer/Controller Medicines

Traditionally, preventer drugs are anti-inflammatory drugs that are either steroids or nonsteroidal. Recently, a new class of drugs called leukotriene agents has been introduced.

What They Do:

As the name suggests, anti-inflammatories help prevent or reduce the underlying inflammation and swelling of your child's air passages. They interrupt the inflammatory process by interfering with the release of cytokines, chemicals that initiate the inflammatory process. They help make the air passages less twitchy and less sensitive to triggers. They must be taken every day, whether your child has symptoms or not, to help prevent attacks. They will not stop an attack once it has started.

Corticosteroids are the most often used preventer medications. They are most commonly inhaled, and this form must be used on a regular basis to be effective. Inhaled corticosteroids include beclomethasone (Beclovent, Vanceril); triamcinolone (Azmacort); flunisolide (AeroBid); and fluticasone. Alternatively, corticosteroids are also taken for short periods of time as tablets or syrups when air passages are very swollen, or if your child has a viral infection. Swallowed corticosteroids include prednisone (Deltasone); methylprednisolone (Medrol); and prednisolone (Prelone, Pediapred).

Side Effects: Possible effects of inhaled corticosteroids include hoarseness, dry mouth, fungal infection of the mouth, and headache. We recommend that you teach your child to use a spacer and rinse his mouth out with water after inhaling the medication to reduce the likelihood of side effects. Possible side effects of swallowed corticosteroids are acne, weight gain, mood changes, stomach upset, high blood pressure, eye problems, and bone problems. The longer the medication is used, the more the possibility of serious side effects. In addition, if these medications are stopped abruptly, problems can occur. The *Journal of the American Medical Association* reported in March 1997 that long-term use of corticosteroids greatly increases the risk of glaucoma, the leading cause of blindness.

Inhaled steroids may also increase the risk of cataracts by 50 percent, according to a study published in the July 3, 1997, issue of the *New England Journal of Medicine*. Recent data also indicate that high doses of these drugs may interfere with sex hormone production and lead to bone loss; they also suppress the adrenal glands and hence may stunt growth. Over the short term, inhaled steroids can cause mood swings and behavior problems, increase the risk of thrush (candida overgrowth), and cause difficulty in speaking.

Nonsteroidals is another class of drugs that inhibit inflammation; they help protect the airways from allergens and they may also help prevent attacks provoked by exercise. They are less effective than steroids, but they are often prescribed for children because they are safer. Nonsteroidals are inhaled and must be used regularly to reduce attacks. The most commonly used nonsteroidal for treating asthma is nedocromil (Tilade).

Side Effects: Rare; dry throat, bad taste in mouth, and nausea.

Sodium cromolyn is a type of medication that stops mast cells from releasing histamine, reducing the sensitivity of the airways. However, unlike antihistamine medications, sodium cromolyn does not block the formation of histamine; rather, it blocks the effects of histamine on the respiratory system cells. Sodium cromolyn is not as drying to the respiratory passages as antihistamines. This is the medication that we prefer to use because it is effective, yet the side effects are minimal; in fact, we recommend the herb from which this drug is derived (ammi visnaga) in our herbal program (see Chapter 7). We have seen excellent results when we prescribe this drug for exercise-induced asthma. Cromolyn needs to be taken regularly to see results. The brand name for cromolyn is Intal.

Side Effects: Rare or none.

Long-Acting Bronchodilators work slowly, but are active over a longer period of time than quick-acting bronchodilators used as reliever medications. They need to be used regularly and are particularly useful in preventing attacks that occur due to exercise or during the night, but will not help an attack once it has started. These medications may be inhaled or swallowed. The commonly used inhalant is salmeterol (Serevent). Other long-acting bronchodilators which are swallowed include theophylline (Slo-bid, Slo-Phyllin, Somophyllin, Theo-Dur, and Uniphyl).

Side Effects: These include headache; dizziness; insomnia; irritability; nervousness; muscle twitching; faster heartbeat; and nausea, vomiting, or diarrhea. Other more serious side effects, such as seizures, may occur if you exceed the amount prescribed. Blood drug levels may be monitored as a preventive measure.

Leukotriene inhibitors are the first new class of asthma drugs in twenty years. They block the action of leukotrienes, the inflammatory chemicals produced by inflammatory cells. The first to be approved by the Food and Drug Administration are called zafirklukast (Accolate), for children twelve and older and montelukast (Zyflo), for children six years of age and older.

Side effects: Headache, infection, and nausea are the most common.

Reliever/Rescue Medicines

These are brochodilators and include beta-agonists and anticholinergics. There is also a short-acting theophylline, which may be used in some cases as a reliever medicine.

What They Do:

These medications bring quick relief. They make breathing easier by temporarily relaxing the muscles around the air passages, allowing the passage to widen (dilate). Bronchodilators used as reliever medications are short-acting and help stop or prevent attacks, depending on the medication. They are usually inhaled, but are also available as syrups.

Beta-agonists are related to adrenaline and are the most powerful and rapid type of reliever medications. They are usually used to stop episodes in progress, but also may be used to prevent flare-ups triggered by exercise. Common medications of this type are albuterol (Ventolin, Proventil); terbutaline (Brethine); metaproterenol (Alupent, Metaprel); bitolterol (Tornalate); and pirbuterol (Maxair).

Side Effects: The most frequently seen effects are shakiness; hyperactivity; nervousness; dizziness; tremors; headache; insomnia; and irregular, pounding, or faster heartbeat. These medications generally should not be taken more than four times a day.

Anticholinergics also relax the bronchial muscles but take longer to act than beta-agonists. They are usually used along with beta-agonists to achieve greater relaxation than beta-agonists achieve alone. The most common type of this medication is ipratropium (Atrovent).

Side Effects: Side effects are rare and are mainly dry mouth and throat.

USING MEDICATIONS WISELY

Using medications improperly can prevent them from helping your child and may increase the risk of harmful side effects. Make sure your child knows how to take asthma medication correctly. According to Dr. Henry Milgrom of Denver's National Jewish Medical and Research Center, only 50 percent of inhaled medication is taken as prescribed. According to several studies, the situation may be worse; they show that 70 to 80 percent of people who use metered-dose inhalers do not use them correctly and thus do not get all the benefits. Discuss with your doctor the types of drugs your child is using and the proper use of an inhaler (a pocket-sized device that releases a quick puff of medication), a spacer (a device that is attached to an inhaler in order to channel the medication more effectively into the lungs), and a nebulizer (a larger device with an air pump that delivers medication over a longer period of time, via a mask placed over the mouth and nose).

Today, children are often taking both preventer drugs (on a regular basis) and reliever drugs (intermittently, as needed). These are also given in the emergency room, in larger doses, when your child has life-threatening symptoms. As a parent, you need to be aware of how your child reacts to drugs so you can make sure he is getting the best care. Jimmy's mother, who had to educate herself about asthma drugs, recalls her experiences with theophylline. "In addition to prednisone, he was getting what they call theophylline 'sprinkles'—a powder you sprinkle on apple juice. I came to realize that this drug all but made Jimmy psychotic, he was completely out of it, he didn't even recognize me. When given too much too fast, he also gets sick to his stomach and throws up. One time, they did give him too much, and he threw up all over the emergency room. So now, I say: Do not give him theophylline, or give him the minimum dosage and wait to see how he reacts." Thankfully, theophylline is given less and less frequently to children because there are other drugs that may be just as effective and pose less risk of side effects.

The Problem with Conventional Asthma Medications

For some children, conventional medications make the difference between playing catch with their friends and staying home; for others they can mean the difference between life and death. Unfortunately, such asthma medications are not the whole answer. At best, they are an imperfect solution. They are a form of crisis treatment—even so-called preventer anti-inflammatory medications *suppress* inflammation rather than encourage the body's natural healing processes. They may prevent an episode, but they do not prevent the underlying conditions in the body that lead to the episode.

Furthermore, they add to the toxic load, making your child's kidneys, liver, and immune system organs work overtime. Steroids are known to deplete the body of important nutrients (potassium, magnesium, and calcium); they suppress immune function, which may increase your child's risk of infection (infection can trigger asthma).

What's more, their undesirable effects—especially long-term effects such as increased risk of glaucoma and bone deterioration—are troubling. This is why in standard medical practice steroids are considered to be appropriate only for children with moderate to severe cases of the disorder. But many physicians have been prescribing them more aggressively, especially in children, on the theory that this might prevent inflammation and keep the disease from getting worse. Dr. Fernando Martinez, professor of pediatrics at the University of Arizona and a member of the expert panel that issued the glaucoma report, is one of a growing number of physicians who have reservations about this practice. He feels that "based on the data in adults, doctors have increasingly believed that we should start using these inhaled steroids earlier and earlier because perhaps we could change the natural course of the disease. . . . My fear is that we don't yet know what the safety profile is for these medicines." Many doctors—and parents—are thus caught in a bind. By giving children high doses of anti-inflammatory steroids to prevent asthma episodes today, they may inadvertently be increasing the children's risk of blindness or a broken hip at a relatively early age.

As you'll see in subsequent chapters, there are safer alternatives to using steroids to reduce inflammation. For example, eliminating certain foods such as peanuts and milk and adding certain nutritional supplements such as vitamins C and E and beta-carotene, quercetin, omega–3 fatty acids, and bioflavonoids can dampen the inflammatory process that your child may now be using steroids to control. Natural medicine offers safer alternative treatments for reliever drugs as well; for example, magnesium supplements and certain herbs can relax the bronchi.

Some final reasons to avoid depending solely on conventional medicines is that they may not always be available during an flare-up. They tend to foster dependence and a "sickly child" mentality that hampers living a normal life. Conventional medications can eventually lose their potency, until even higher and higher doses fail to stop symptoms completely. What happens if the medicine is used so often it stops working?

What About Other Medicines?

Allergies and colds are frequent asthma triggers. When your child suffers from either one, you may tempted to ease symptoms with conventional prescription or nonprescription medications. As is the case with asthma medications, these will suppress symptoms, add to your child's toxic burden, and may cause side effects. We recommend that you carefully consider using the following medications, and use them only as a last resort after trying the natural remedies suggested in this book:

Antihistamines: These include Benadryl, Tavist, Chlor-Trimeton, and Zyrtec. They offer relief for itchy, watery eyes, sneezing, runny nose, swollen throat, and hives. These act as sedatives, and side effects include drowsiness; impaired coordination; dry mouth, nose, and throat; and insomnia after stopping medication. Newer antihistamines such as Claritin, Allegra, and Hismanal cause less drowsiness. Antihistamines should not be used during an acute asthma episode because they cause mucus to dry up—and when that happens, the airways become narrower which in turn worsens asthma symptoms.

Oral Decongestants: These include Sudafed, Tylenol Sinus, and Sine-Aid. They offer relief for stuffy nose.

These act as stimulants, and their side effects include elevated blood pressure; increased heart rate; nervousness; insomnia.

Nasal Decongestants: These include Afrin and Vicks Sinex. They offer relief for stuffy nose. They also act as stimulants, and their main side effect is rebound stuffiness—symptoms can worsen with prolonged use of sprays.

Antihistamine/Decongestants: These include Actifed, Tavist-D, and Sinutab. They offer relief for itchy, watery eyes, sneezing, runny nose, swollen throat, and stuffy nose. They are often used preventively to avoid allergic reactions that can trigger asthma. Some antihistamines dilate the bronchial tubes, but most of the symptom relief comes from their ability to block the production of histamine, the most potent inflammatory chemical in the body. Antihistamines enable your child to breathe through his nose, rather than his mouth, and this warms and humidifies air, which reduces the likelihood of irritation, coughing, and asthma. They act as both sedatives and stimulants, and side effects therefore include restlessness and/or drowsiness.

Antibiotics: It is widely acknowledged that antibiotics, which kill bacteria, are overused and misused, particularly for colds and flu, which are caused by viruses. Antibiotics are even more liberally prescribed for children with asthma because upper respiratory infections are a common trigger for asthma symptoms. Yet these drugs can add to your child's toxic burden, compromise the immune system, and worsen asthma problems. Antibiotics, which are also often given to children, can create an imbalance in the body and

lead to an overgrowth of yeast. That's why, when your child
has an upper respiratory infection, we feel the best course is
to use natural therapies to bolster your child's immune system so minor viral and bacterial infections stay minor and go
away quickly. With the appropriate natural care, a cold or
flu can leave her immune system in better shape, and she is
less likely to suffer complications.

As you'll see in subsequent chapters, natural medicine offers
many nontoxic ways to prevent and manage colds, flu, and allergies.

THE ROLE OF NATURAL MEDICINE

Since asthma can be a life-threatening disease, our philosophy is
that conventional asthma medications have their place. But as
with any disease, *prevention is preferable to treatment*. Although
drugs may sometimes be necessary, they do nothing to reduce the
toxic burden that is the underlying cause of the inflammation that
leads to symptoms of asthma—on the contrary, they *add to* the
toxic burden. In fact, studies show that taking asthma medicine on
a regular basis can actually contribute to symptoms of asthma and
increase the risk of a flare-up.

What Our Natural Asthma
Control Program Has to Offer

Basing medical care on natural therapies, on the other hand,
effectively *reduces the toxic burden*. The approaches we use in our
practice include general lifestyle changes, diet and nutritional supplementation, herbs and homeopathy, acupuncture and acupressure,
and psychological therapies. We have found that such approaches

minimize the exposure to toxins including those in air, food, water, antibiotics, and anti-asthma drugs, as well as strengthen a child's constitution so he reacts less severely to whatever toxins cannot be avoided—including conventional drugs when necessary—and resists infections that can trigger asthma.

Our program recognizes that asthma is both a physical condition and a highly charged emotional issue. Contrary to popular belief, asthma is not psychosomatic, and science is gradually beginning to understand the true relationship between the mind and body and how this relates specifically to asthma. Certainly emotional stresses can contribute to or worsen an episode, and we give you the practical tools to cope with whatever stresses are triggering your child's flare-ups. But scientific thinking has shifted its attention to the emotional fallout of coping with asthma, which is considerable. It is clear to us that there are such things as "toxic emotions"—negative thoughts and feelings that can affect the immune system and, hence, the course of the illness. This is why we emphasize ways for you to identify toxic emotions and learn the coping skills needed by the whole family to detoxify their relationships and their children's emotional environment. We also supply specific mind-body therapies that the child, parent, and whole family can learn to use to nip stress in the bud.

Natural medicines can be used for prevention by treating the chronic aspect and for symptom relief during an acute episode. They can be used for preventing and relieving triggers such as colds and allergies, which ultimately also help to prevent asthma. In summary, our program:

- helps prevent asthmatic episodes by slowing and calming down the chronic inflammation caused by chronic toxic overload;

- relieves symptoms by relaxing the airways during non-life-threatening episodes—without harmful side effects;
- reduces the need for conventional drugs, making them safer and more effective to use under appropriate circumstances;
- gives the body what it needs to heal itself, avoid permanent lung damage, and encourage healthy new lung tissue to grow;
- improves the child's quality of life now and during adulthood;
- minimizes emergency room visits, time lost from school, and time lost from work, reducing anxiety and saving money in the process;
- addresses the emotional aspects of asthma for the child and the whole family.

Natural Medicine Is Worth the Effort

Time and time again, our patients say that integrating natural therapies into an asthma control program is worth it. Natural medicine may cost extra and take more time initially, but it ultimately will save you money, time, effort, and anguish. Asthma can be enormously expensive when you calculate the costs over the lifetime of your child. You need to pay for medication, doctor visits, hospital stays, emergency room treatments, and time off from work when you care for your child. Insurance helps pay, of course, but rarely 100 percent. The least expensive way to control asthma is to get at the underlying cause—the problem of chronic inflammation caused by toxic overload.

Instead of unwanted side effects, the natural therapies suggested here often have more than one beneficial effect. In implementing this program, you are instilling in your child good health habits and an integrated approach to medicine that he or she will carry through life. In the process, you are not only taking care of asthma, but safeguarding your child's overall health by reducing the risk factors for a slew of other diseases, including cancer, heart disease, osteoporosis, and diabetes.

Yes, this program is more work than relying on reliever drugs, and yes, the family has to take responsibility and make an effort. However, the extra effort is worth the investment.

Remember, you don't have to do it all at once, and it's not an all-or-nothing situation. We designed this program so you can individualize it and use as few as two or three approaches—or as many as all seven. Once you begin, you can tailor it further, and vary it depending on your child's response and the circumstances. One thing is etched in stone: By taking the positive health-building actions in our program you will feel less helpless, more empowered, more in control, more self-reliant, and your child will gradually feel and do better and better.

THREE — PREPARING FOR THE PROGRAM

Asthma is a serious condition and can get more serious as time goes on. We feel strongly that to ensure success you need to prepare your child, yourself, and your family before making any changes in your child's current treatment plan. We understand that you are eager to begin, but recommend that you first lay a firm foundation.

Use this chapter as a checklist to make sure you are prepared to take this big step: Do you have the kind of doctor you can work with? We explain why your child needs the most experienced, qualified medical care you can find and give you our opinion as to what kind of doctor can best provide it. Do you know how asthma is diagnosed and evaluated? We explain the standard procedures of a conventional diagnosis as well as the pros and cons of consulting an allergist for allergy testing. Are you ready psychologically for the changes you will be making? At the end of this chapter, we offer a pep talk to get you motivated and ready to begin the program that starts in Chapter 4.

FINDING THE RIGHT PHYSICIAN

Your child is probably already under a doctor's care—but is he or she the right doctor? The safest and most effective way to follow the

Natural Asthma Control Program is under the care of a physician who is knowledgeable about childhood asthma, allergies, and sensitivities, and who can treat these conditions with natural therapies.

Of course, it is possible to patch together a team of health care practitioners consisting of a conventional physician who has an open mind about natural therapies plus a naturopathic physician, nutritionist, herbalist, or homeopath. If you need to follow this route, we recommend you look for a naturopath because he or she will be able to provide a broader spectrum of therapies than a practitioner who specializes in any one field. You will find sources for alternative health practitioners in the Resources section of this book; locate one in your geographic area and work closely with them within their area of expertise. Again, this is not ideal, but it may be your best option if you live in certain areas of the country.

We strongly feel that the ideal situation is to find someone who can do it all—a medical doctor who can diagnose and evaluate your child, prescribe conventional asthma medications, help you monitor the severity and frequency of symptoms, provide a well-thought-out treatment plan, consult with you during emergencies, *and* use natural therapies.

The type of medicine this kind of physician practices goes under several names—holistic, integrative, or progressive medicine. This is the form of medicine we practice at our centers in Rhinebeck and Albany; we prefer the terms "progressive medicine" and "progressive physician." This form of medicine involves blending the best that conventional and natural therapies have to offer. Often, when patients come to us they have gone the conventional route and are dissatisfied with the results; perhaps they have tried some natural therapies but their knowledge was incomplete and they were disappointed with the results. But when the two forms of medicine are combined correctly, they are amazed at the results—their children suffer fewer and milder symptoms and flare-ups are rare or nonexistent. And they don't experience the stress, confusion, and lack of information, advice, and coordination inherent in working with a doctor who knows nothing about natural therapies—or worse, is antagonistic.

Diane's mother had a typical experience with a conventional physician. She says, "All he did was give albuterol for her asthma and antibiotics for her constant ear infections. In a two-year-old, the side effects from these things were terrible—rashes, diarrhea—it's worse than the disease. I tried to talk to him about her allergies, her medication, but I never got anything back from him—he didn't want to hear, he didn't seem to care. But when I talk to Dr. Bock, he listens, he talks back to you, nothing you say is too far-fetched. It was a huge relief to find someone who made us aware of what was going on with Diane, and I felt safe because he offers all these natural therapies, but he's a physician too."

Another criterion for choosing a physician is less tangible but no less important. It is always preferable to have a physician who, in addition to having technical expertise, is someone with whom you and your child are comfortable. It is particularly important to find a doctor with whom you and your child have good chemistry, because this is a chronic disease that requires ongoing and highly individualized care, and because there is a strong psychological component to the condition and its treatment. Is there trust and good communication between your doctor and you and your child? Does the doctor give you the time you need to have your questions and concerns addressed? Is he or she interested in working with you to reduce medication through natural methods?

Whether you see a family physician (also called a general practitioner, primary care physician, or internist) or a pediatrician, we strongly urge you to find a progressive physician who practices integrated medicine. Like us, more and more physicians are embracing the best of both worlds and offering them to their patients in a responsible, caring, scientifically responsible way. If you are seeing a doctor who is sympathetic to natural therapies but does not offer them himself, you will be getting fragmented care. This is still an improvement over conventional care only, but is not ideal. Even if you cannot find physicians like us who specialize in allergies and asthma, a progressive physician can still orchestrate the treatments offered by practitioners specializing in particular therapies, such as herbalists or nutritionists, and supervise the reduction of conventional medicine as your child's condition improves.

If your current doctor doesn't meet these criteria, or is openly antagonistic to natural therapies, it is worth trying to find one who will make success more likely by being supportive, sympathetic, and willing to try something new.

As with any condition, the most common way to find a doctor is through recommendation. Ask your current doctor, friends, relatives, and acquaintances if they know a physician who might be appropriate. Check with the American College for Advancement in Medicine (ACAM), the American Academy of Environmental Medicine, and the American Holistic Medicine Association (see listings in the "Resources" section of this book). You may also want to call several of the growing number of medical schools that offer programs in complementary medicine and will provide you with a list of their graduates with practices in your geographical area. According to an article published in 1998 in the *Journal of the American Medical Association*, more than half of the medical schools in the United States now offer courses that include alternative medicines such as homeopathy, herbal therapy, and mind-body techniques. This is wonderful news for people who, as the researchers note, "are increasingly seeking to identify a physician who is solidly grounded in conventional, orthodox medicine and is also knowledgeable about the value and limitations of alternative treatment." However, they caution that this does not mean that all courses are created equal—the survey found a tremendous diversity in the content, format, and course requirements, and the researchers believe "the development of a more consistent educational approach to this provocative area is essential." So, you still need to shop carefully and ask questions about the qualifications and training of any prospective physician. And unfortunately, with managed care, you may not always get the doctor of your choice, or get the continuity of care that your child needs.

The Diagnosis

This may seem obvious, but you need to make sure that your child actually has asthma and find out how severe it is. Many other conditions can mimic asthma and require different treatment; an exam can help rule these out. Getting a professional diagnosis is a key part of preparing for this program.

The most important part of the exam is a detailed medical history. The doctor will want to know your child's symptoms, how often they occur, when they occur, and whether anything seems to trigger, aggravate, or alleviate symptoms. You may be asked about your child's home and school environment and about other activities. It can be difficult to be accurate and objective when retelling your child's history; that's why writing down your child's symptoms before the doctor's visit, using the charts and forms provided in the next chapter, can be invaluable.

The doctor will also give your child a physical exam which focuses on the upper airways and lungs for signs and symptoms of asthma. He or she may listen to your child's breathing through a stethoscope and examine your child's nose, ears, eyes, and throat for signs of allergies.

When appropriate the doctor will order tests, including a chest X-ray to rule out other diseases and to detect any complications, such as pneumonia; certain blood tests; and a lung function test. This test uses a device called a spirometer to measure the air flowing in and out of your child's lungs. However, there is no lab test that definitively confirms a diagnosis of asthma. Sometimes the definitive diagnosis is made by giving a coughing or wheezing child asthma medication and noting whether this improves symptoms. If it does, the diagnosis of asthma is confirmed.

Once asthma has been diagnosed, your child's doctor should give you a written plan that tells you exactly what medications to take, when to take them, and the proper dose. As explained in the next chapter, the plan is usually divided into three zones, which are part of a continuum. The green zone means the asthma is under control and that you should continue with the current medication plan. The yellow zone signifies mild asthma symptoms—you need to modify the medication. The red zone indicates that symptoms are worsening and that you should call your doctor immediately or seek emergency medical treatment.

SHOULD YOU SEE AN ALLERGIST?

In the following chapter, we provide you with a self-assessment that will help you detect allergies and other triggers of your child's asthma. If allergies are a strong component in your child's asthma, you need to address this. Your primary physician may have clinical experience or have an expertise in allergies, as we do. If not, consider getting a referral to an allergist from your doctor. If your child's allergies seem to be complex, a conservative and often helpful approach would be to see an allergist who is certified by the American Board of Allergy and Clinical Immunology. However, a clinical ecologist who is a member of the American Academy of Environmental Medicine will also be able to handle most allergies. This type of physician takes a broader view of what causes allergies and sensitivities and may be able to detect problems that a more conservative approach would not.

Time and time again, our patients have said that their previous doctors did not find any allergies, or didn't "believe" that food allergies could cause asthma. Yet when we tested their children, we often found hidden allergies. And when their children avoided these newly diagnosed allergens, they improved remarkably.

Testing for Allergies

There are many ways an allergist will try to more accurately pinpoint the allergens that provoke your child's symptoms. These include:

A scratch test in which the doctor makes several scratches on the surface of your child's skin and then applies the suspected allergens to the abraded area to see if any of them show a reaction.

An intradermal test in which the allergens are applied a bit more deeply under the skin.

RAST blood tests which look for elevated levels of specific immunoglobulins. In our practice, we have found that testing the blood for IgE is an effective way to detect allergies to inhaled allergens and to detect one-third of food allergies; testing for IgG, another immunoglobulin, detects the other two-thirds of food allergies. RAST stands for radioallergosorbent tests.

Treating Allergies

If your child is allergic, you have a wide array of treatment choices. The first and foremost step to take is to *avoid allergens*. We discuss this at length in Chapter 5. However, you can't always avoid all allergens. Therefore, we sometimes treat allergies with:

Antihistamines. Conventional antihistamines have their limitations, as explained in Chapter 2. We prefer to use natural antihistamines such as nutritional supplements, herbs, and homeopathy.

Allergy shots (immunotherapy). Immunotherapy, though controversial for asthma, may be helpful if your child is allergic to substances that are hard to avoid; the allergy shots can take several months to a year or more to start working.

Antiyeast therapy. In many cases, our patients are suffering from an overgrowth of yeast, the most common type of which is called *candida albicans*. This overgrowth affects the immune system and increases its sensitivity, making a child more likely to be allergic to foods, chemicals, and inhaled allergens. We treat this condition with a special diet and antiyeast medication.

Enzyme-Potentiated Desensitiziation (EPD). We have had good results with this form of immunotherapy in our patients with inhalant allergies as well as food and chemical allergies and sensitivities. In this technique, we combine extremely small doses of allergens with the enzyme beta-glucuronidase. This enzyme potentiates (increases) the desired immune response. For a list of physicians who offer EPD in your area, send a stamped, self-addressed envelope to the American EPD Society, 141 Pasea de Paralta, Santa Fe, New Mexico 87501; phone 505–983–8890; fax 505–820–7315. Be sure to specify the names of the state you live in and the surrounding states.

Nambudripad Allergy Elimination Technique (NAET). This is an exciting new technique developed by Devi Nambudripad, Ph.D., a registered nurse, licensed acupuncturist, and chiropractor. NAET combines the principles of Chinese medicine and chiropractic to identify allergens and then clear the body of its allergic response to those substances. Because we have seen very impressive results in patients we refer to NAET practitioners, we have incorporated this approach in our clinic. The advantage to this technique is that it reprograms the nervous system so it stops overreacting to the allergens. Once your child has been treated, he needs to avoid the allergen for twenty-five hours, and after that he is no longer allergic. To find out more about this technique, and for a listing of practitioners in your state, go to the Web site www.allergy2000.com, or buy the book, *Winning the War Against Asthma & Allergies* by Ellen W. Cutler, D.C., Delmar Publishers, 1997. Or you can contact our clinic.

WHAT ABOUT YOUR OTHER CHILDREN?

In many children, symptoms of asthma are subtle. If one of your children has been diagnosed with asthma, your other children are at higher risk of having asthma too. Suspect asthma if:

- your child has colds that cause him or her to cough more than other children;
- the cough continues for weeks after the cold has gone away;
- colds always seem to "settle" in the chest, rather than cause primarily nasal congestion.

To prevent asthma from developing in another child, we advise that you minimize your child's exposure to the triggers discussed in Chapter 5, and to minimize the likelihood of the child developing food allergies, as suggested in Chapter 6. Even prenatal exposure to allergens can increase the risk of asthma, so it's best if you avoid them while pregnant.

A PEP TALK:
GETTING PSYCHED UP

We recognize that it takes courage to begin this program. Asthma is unlike other childhood illnesses. Nothing compares with the powerlessness and frustration you feel when your child is struggling for air. You want and need to *do something*. We have seen how difficult it is for parents to trust that they are doing the right thing by trying alternative therapy. They are under a tremendous amount of internal pressure and pressure from others, including conventional pediatricians and friends and other family members.

We want to reassure you that our program is based on the latest scientific evidence and the thirty years of collective experience that we have in treating childhood asthma. We know that this approach works, and our seasoned patients know it too. But since one of us (Steve) has spent the early part of his career as an emergency room physician, we also know the terror that can paralyze parents and keep them clinging to the life raft of conventional medicine. Part of you wants to get at the root cause of asthma and wean your child away from conventional drugs, but the thought of taking away your child's medication may also be frightening. You may ask yourself now and then: Am I doing the right thing? Only you can answer this question. As you gain experience and confidence, as you see your child getting better, the more easily you'll be able to say yes.

You will find it especially challenging to make these life changes if your friends, family, and doctor are skeptical and nonsupportive. Be sure to show them this book so they can educate themselves. Rest assured that there are other parents all over the country who have used natural therapies. Some of them share their fears and eventual triumphs with you in the final chapter of this book. You may also want to turn to support groups and chat rooms available on the Internet, through Mothers of Asthmatics, and through your local chapter of the American Lung Association. They are wonderful sources for empathy and psychological support.

Remember that teamwork eases your burden and makes the program more successful. Just as no single therapy is the sole solution, no one person is the sole caregiver. You can't do it alone—you need the cooperation and contributions of your child, spouse, primary physician, natural medicine practitioner, and nurses. For advice about involving your child and school personnel in the program, please turn to Chapter 9, "Living Well with Asthma."

Watching what you eat, taking supplements, and using herbs are becoming more common. We live in an age when Oprah publicly eschews meat and homeopathic remedies are sold in chain drugstores. This climate makes it easier than ever before to follow our natural program. It also makes it easier for you to downplay your child's asthma as the reason for your lifestyle changes. So when the going gets tough, remind yourself: you are doing more than helping your child control asthma naturally. You are also helping him control allergies, reduce the incidence of colds and flu, and benefiting his health in other ways so he can live a normal, happy, productive life. And if you and your family follow the program, everyone will enjoy better overall health.

FOUR

HOW TO USE OUR PROGRAM

In the previous chapter we explained *why* it's better for your child when you integrate natural therapies into an asthma control program. Now the question is *how* to do it. In this chapter, we provide you with a road map that is similar to the personalized guidance we give the parents of our patients.

To begin, we show you how to establish a monitoring system to guide you and your doctor in safely reducing your child's asthma medication. This process should take about one month. We then show you how to gradually create a holistic program tailored to the needs of your child and family; since each child and situation is unique, for this phase we will show you how to create your own timetable.

ACTION STEP:

DOCUMENT THE
LONG-TERM HISTORY

Before you can change something, you need to know where you stand now. So, the first step you take to launch the program is to document the history of your child's asthma. To do this, pull together a long-term picture of at least one year, and preferably up to three years—the duration depends on the age of your child and the onset of symptoms or date of diagnosis. Record your child's doctor visits, emergency room visits, and hospitalizations; the medications he or she has been taking; and the other illnesses. If you use the chart provided on page 55, make one photocopy of the blank chart for each year of record. Fill in the blanks, using all available medical records (you may need to get some information from your doctor), and also call upon your memories and those of other family members, placing an X or shading in the area under the month to indicate the time periods as accurately as possible.

This record will provide valuable information for you, your child's primary physician, and any natural health care practitioner whom you choose. The history gives a glimpse back in time and allows you to spot overall trends and patterns—is your child getting worse or better? Do episodes tend to occur in the spring, which may indicate allergies to pollen? Are they more frequent in the winter, when he catches colds?

ACTION STEP:

USING THE ZONES TO ESTABLISH A MONITORING SYSTEM

The next step is to have in place a means of following your child's condition. Your doctor has of course been monitoring your child's condition every time you visit the medical office. Most likely he or she has also advised you about the best way to monitor your child's condition at home. Under conventional treatment, monitoring your child allows you to gauge what medication she should be taking to control symptoms if they occur, help prevent sudden severe flare-ups, help your child maintain a normal level of activity, and tell you whether to seek professional care. Under this program, monitoring allows you to do that and more: It allows you to

LONG TERM MEDICAL HISTORY

Child's name: _____ Year: _____

Doctor's name(s): _____

	Jan	Feb	Mar	Apr	May	Jun	Jul	Aug	Sep	Oct	Nov	Dec
Doctor's Visits												

Comments

	Jan	Feb	Mar	Apr	May	Jun	Jul	Aug	Sep	Oct	Nov	Dec
Hospitalizations												

Comments

	Jan	Feb	Mar	Apr	May	Jun	Jul	Aug	Sep	Oct	Nov	Dec
Asthma Medications												

Name of medication
Side effects

Name of medication
Side effects

Name of medication
Side effects

Other Illnesses

Comments

Other Medications

work with your doctor in judging when it is safe to begin reducing your child's use of medication.

Most asthma treatment plans involve categorizing symptoms and peak flow levels according to three *zones*. In our program, you will also use these three zones, which are explained below. The zones take into consideration two ways of monitoring: observing your child's symptoms and using a device called a peak flow meter.

Monitoring by observing your child's symptoms.

Use this method for your child, no matter how old he is. This is an effective, "low-tech" way to check on your child's condition, regardless of age. However, in young children, observing symptoms is the only way you can tell how your child is faring. Being familiar with the symptoms is important in preventing and treating severe episodes. To determine which zone your child is in at any particular time, compare your child's current symptoms with the symptoms listed in the zones.

Monitoring using a peak flow meter.

This method works for older children only. It requires using a peak flow meter, an easy-to-read, simple device that measures the speed at which your child can push air out of her lungs and thus reliably indicates how open her airways are. A peak flow reading is more objective and accurate than relying on observing signs and symptoms alone. It lets you know more precisely how well your child is controlling her asthma and gives advance notice of a possible flare-up—even before there are noticeable symptoms.

Bear in mind that peak flow meters are most successfully used in children seven years of age and older; between the ages of four and six it is difficult to use this device; and in children under four they are quite unreliable. It's likely that your child's doctor has already prescribed a peak flow meter. If not, we encourage every parent whose child is seven or older to buy and use a peak flow meter and use it regularly—in the morning, the evening, after exposure to a trigger, and when symptoms seem to be worsening.

Make sure that you and your child understand how to use a peak flow meter correctly. After measuring for two to three weeks you will be able to determine your child's *personal best* peak flow reading. This is the highest reading your child can achieve. If your child has chronic symptoms, this level will improve with our program. Write the number here:

Personal Best Peak Flow Reading _____

Date: _____

THE THREE ZONES

These zones are usually called green, yellow, and red zones, similar to a traffic light. The green zone means "all clear—go or continue;" the yellow zone means "caution—slow down;" the red zone means "danger—stop." Your health care practitioner will tell you the various levels of peak flow in your child that correspond to the three categories/zones provided below. To determine which zone your child is in at any particular time, compare your child's current peak flow level with the levels that your health practitioner has given you.

Once you begin the Natural Asthma Control Program, use the symptoms listed in the zones and peak flow readings to give you and your child concrete, positive reinforcement that what you are doing is really helping her control her asthma, and the confidence to wean her away from medication.

GREEN ZONE:
GOOD ASTHMA CONTROL

These are signs that your child is doing well, has minimal inflammation of the airways, and should *continue his or her usual treatment.* Your child's asthma is under good control if he or she:

- rarely or never coughs during the night;
- rarely or never awakens at night because of coughing or shortness of breath;
- actively plays with other children with little or no coughing, wheezing, chest tightness, or shortness of breath;
- gets colds of similar severity to other children;
- peak flow reading is: ___ (between 80 and 100 percent of your child's personal best).

YELLOW ZONE:
EARLY WARNING SIGNS

These are signs that your child's asthma may be getting worse and there is increasing swelling and inflammation of the air passages. You need to *change the treatment*, as recommended by your doctor. Your child is heading for a flare-up if he or she:

- coughs frequently at night;
- is restless while trying to fall asleep and wakes up frequently at night with coughing or chest tightness and inability to breathe;
- coughs, wheezes, has chest tightness, and has shortness of breath when playing with other children, or is playing less actively because of symptoms;
- coughs or wheezes even when not physically active
- has an itchy throat;
- has colds that are more frequent, severe, and longer lasting than other children's;
- has unexplained fatigue or mood changes;
- peak flow reading is: ____ (between 50 and 79 percent of your child's personal best).

RED ZONE:
DANGER SIGNS
OF SEVERE
ASTHMA FLARE-UP

These signs indicate an *asthma emergency*. Give your child reliever medication as recommended by your doctor and *call your doctor immediately* or go to the hospital right away. Signs of a severe asthma episode are:

- severe shortness of breath, rapid or shallow breathing, labored breathing, sucking in of the skin between the ribs or at the base of the neck, sits slumped forward with shoulders raised, flared nostrils, difficulty speaking more than a few words between breaths.
- bluish lips or fingers;
- unable to speak in full sentences because of shortness of breath;
- sleepiness and fatigue due to lack of oxygen;
- fainting due to lack of oxygen;
- severe coughing or wheezing that is not relieved by the recommended reliever medication, or symptoms that return within four hours after administering the medication;
- peak flow reading is: _____ (less than 50 percent of your child's personal best).

ACTION STEP:

KEEP A DAILY DIARY

The next step is to begin a daily diary to document the changes so you and your doctor can reduce medication in a logical, safe way.

We recommend that you begin keeping a daily diary for at least two to three weeks before implementing any of the approaches in the Natural Asthma Control Program. This simple task provides you with a structured way to closely observe and get to know your child and become more involved in treating her condition. That way, once you start adding natural therapies, you will be more finely tuned and better able to observe the effects.

Once you begin the program it is absolutely crucial that you continue to keep a daily diary. It is the only way you can confidently, precisely, and completely monitor your child's condition and spot and document trends and patterns of improvement. Thus it is an indispensable tool that lets you know whether you

WHAT TO DO DURING AN ASTHMA FLARE-UP

- Stay calm on the outside, even if you aren't on the inside; take some deep calming breaths yourself.
- Be firm and confident and speak to your child in a reassuring way.
- Give your child the medication agreed upon by you and your child's doctor.
- Make sure your child drinks plenty of water to avoid dehydration and keep the mucus liquid and flowing.
- Figure out what may have triggered the flare-up and remove the trigger if possible, or move your child away from the trigger. This will help stop the triggering process and give your child a chance to recover.

SAMPLE DAILY DIARY

Date _____

Peak flow _____

Symptoms _____

Time of day _____

Location _____

Duration _____

Time of last meal _____

Possible triggers _____

Psychological state _____

Medications taken _____

Dosage

Frequency

Effectiveness

Side effects

Natural therapies _____

Dosage

Frequency

Effectiveness

Side effects

Note: For a more detailed symptom tracking form, see www.Patients-America.com which is also described in our "Resources" section.

can, with your doctor's supervision, reduce your child's medication safely. The diary also helps you communicate more effectively with your child's doctors, helps determine the effects of the medication, the timing, and the dosage so the doctor can fine tune medical treatment, and helps ensure your child is not getting too much or too little medication. It also gives valuable clues to which substances and conditions act as triggers for your child's asthma, which is an advantage when you get to the next chapter.

To keep the diary, use one page of loose-leaf paper per day or a printed daily calendar, or you can buy blank diary pages from Pedipress (see "Resources" section). Place them in your loose-leaf binder along with the medical history. Every day record your child's condition. Describe the symptoms, and include when the symptoms occurred, where your child was at the time, the time of his last meal, the duration of the episode, and make a note of any suspected triggers. Be sure to include the name, amount, and

GETTING ORGANIZED

A loose-leaf binder is the best way to keep all records orderly and in one place for easy reference. Buy one at any stationery store and keep the medical history and daily diary pages in it. The Allergy and Asthma Network sells a product called the Asthma Organizer, a loose-leaf binder system that includes a daily symptoms diary and a variety of other forms to keep track of your child's medications, office visits, and so on. (See "Resources" section.)

frequency of any medications taken, and their effectiveness and side effects. Also record any general comments about his condition and his psychological state—was he feeling any strong emotions at the time? To help you recognize and categorize the symptoms, as well as use consistent terms to refer to them, refer to the earlier section of this chapter which provides you with lists of symptoms in increasing order of severity. If your child is old enough, also enter the peak flow rates. When you begin to add natural therapies, you will also incorporate them into the diary. Take this record with you when visiting your doctor or natural health care practitioner.

ACTION STEP:

START ADDING NATURAL THERAPIES

Once you know where your child stands regarding the intensity and frequency of her asthma symptoms and are comfortable with the monitoring process, you are ready to gradually begin adding the natural therapies presented in the following chapters.

In a nutshell, the program involves gradually introducing natural therapies into your child's existing asthma treatment program. The goal is to stabilize your child's immune system so it is not hyperreactive but powerful and able to resist infection. You continue to monitor your child's symptoms carefully, and when your physician gives you the go-ahead, gradually begin to reduce the use of conventional medications.

Again, we want to emphasize that in this program, you work with your doctor and use natural therapies as complementary therapies *along with* conventional medical treatment. These therapies are compatible with medical treatment, and if you are going to a conventional doctor, your natural health professionals should be able to work with him or her. *Be sure to inform your child's doctor of your intentions and reduce medication only under his or her supervision.*

Tailoring the Program

Since children and family situations differ, this is not a one-size-fits-all program. We will be making suggestions and offering you guidelines, but you will be tailoring your plan to suit your unique situation from the very beginning and continuing to modify the program as your child progresses. Each of the following chapters deals with one specific therapy or approach.

Where to begin?

We recommend that everyone begin by "Avoiding Common Triggers" (Chapter 5), because this is the most effective approach you can take overall, and is the foundation of both conventional and natural asthma therapy. Then in a step-by-step progressive manner, gradually add on elements from the remaining chapters. We recommend you next add "Food as Healer" (Chapter 6), first of all because many foods act as triggers and should be avoided, and second because certain types of foods contain health-building nutrients. Next, we would recommend giving your child "Nutritional Supplements" (Chapter 7), which provide additional health-building nutrients beyond what food contains. After that, you may add "Herbs and Other Plant Remedies" (Chapter 8) if that appeals to you. If you are like most families, you will be grappling with psychological issues and may find the techniques in "Living Well with Asthma" (Chapter 9) helpful; in many instances "Mind-Body Medicine" (Chapter 10) can make a huge impact on the well-being of a child—as well as other members of the family.

We recommend you read through all the chapters on natural therapies so you have a basic understanding of what's involved in each one and the role they can play in a comprehensive asthma control program. Then explain this to your child in terms that he can understand. Bear in mind that the choices you make depend on several factors:

• *Your child's preferences.* One key factor is how willing your child is to go along with the therapy. Some children have no problem giving up certain foods or activities that are triggers and emphasizing others that are not. Others object strenuously to giving up Cap'n Crunch, eating broccoli, or banishing their stuffed animals from their bed. Some can take vitamin supplements without batting an eyelash, while others have trouble swallowing pills.

• *Your philosophy.* Your personal preferences and philosophy may strongly influence your choice of natural therapies. For some parents, homeopathy makes a lot of sense; for others, herbs are the way to go, and so on.

• *Your child's response.* Another factor is how well your child responds to a therapy. Certain herbs may work like a charm in some children and have little or no effect in others. Although some children will do well enough after one or two approaches have been integrated into their lives, often it is a comprehensive, holistic program that works best, especially if their asthma is severe. That is because when used together these approaches support each other and have a synergistic effect. We recommend that you add one therapy at a time and give it enough time to judge the results. Then, add the next and then the next. Once your child achieves good control, and maintains this even after you have been able to reduce your use of conventional medicines, then you can start reducing your use of natural therapies as well. As you will see in Chapter 12, once their health has been restored, our patients are able to eat a more "normal" diet, take fewer nutritional supplements, and so on, as time goes by. When you have reached this happy state, we advise that you start cutting down the form of natural therapy that you and your child have found the most difficult to do.

Achieving Your Goals

Since there are two types of medications—preventers and relievers—from which to wean your child, there are two goals to this program.

- *Goal #1: Prevent Asthma Flare-ups.* You can use natural therapies on an ongoing basis to avoid episodes in the first place by reducing the toxic burden, healing the underlying condition, and relieving chronic inflammation and hypersensitivity. If your child is on preventer medication, you may be able to use natural therapies to reduce or replace the need for *preventer medications.*

- *Goal #2: Relieve Symptoms.* You may use natural therapies on an as-needed basis to reduce inflammation and relax the bronchial tubes during a mild worsening of symptoms. In this case, you may be able to use natural therapies to reduce or replace the need for *reliever medications.*

In our practice we first aim for Goal #1 and try to reduce and eventually eliminate preventer medication, and we reserve reliever medications for flare-ups. Since natural therapies can dramatically reduce the frequency and severity of episodes, this may be your only goal. However, we often then progress to Goal #2 and have patients first turn to natural remedies for symptom relief even during a flare-up.

When You Can Reduce Medication:

For our patients, we begin reducing medication when the child has reached the green zone and has remained there for one month, meaning she has achieved the hallmarks of good asthma control and her peak flow reading is at least 80 percent of her personal best, as described on pages 57–58. You should discuss medication reduction with your doctor when your child has improved to this level, unless your doctor advises you otherwise.

Remember if natural remedies are not effective enough, you can always turn to conventional reliever medications. Even if your child has achieved superb control and natural remedies are effective for those rare instances when he has a flare-up, we recommend that you always keep conventional reliever medicine on hand, just in case. Asthma is a serious condition, and you never know when you will confront a powerful trigger that requires the dramatic relief that conventional medicine can provide.

Just as with conventional medicines, you may need to step up the program during certain times of the year or under certain conditions when your child is exposed to more triggers, for example, in the spring if he suffers from hay-fever-type allergies, or in the winter if colds and flu are a trigger for him.

Action Steps to Achieving Goal #1: Prevent Asthma Flare-ups

1: Begin the first form of natural therapy, avoiding common triggers, while continuing preventer medication(s) if any and keeping a daily diary.

2: After one month, use the diary to assess any improvements in your child's condition.

3: If there is some improvement, continue with this therapy until your child is in the green zone. If there is no improvement, continue for one more month. If there is still no improvement, add another natural therapy and assess her condition again after one month. Repeat this process, adding on therapies, until your child reaches the green zone. If you still do not see any progress, consider working with one or more professionals with expertise in natural therapies until your child reaches the green zone.

4: Continue with the program until your child has remained in the green zone for one month.

5: Make an appointment with your child's doctor; bring the daily diary as documentation of her improvement and discuss with the doctor the advisability of reducing your child's preventer medication.

6: If her medication is reduced and she remains in the green zone for a month, as documented in the daily diary, discuss with your doctor the advisability of reducing the medication further.

7: Keep reducing her medication under the doctor's supervision until your child no longer requires it to stay in the green zone for at least one month. If your child leaves the green zone for more than two days of the month, go back to the previous level of medication and try adding one or more natural therapies, as in Step 3, until she is back in the green zone for a month.

Steps to Achieving Goal #2:
Relieve Symptoms

1: If your child's asthma is under good control but on occasion shows mild or moderate worsening of symptoms, you may try a natural remedy to relieve them. Refer to the chapters on individual therapies for specific remedies and dosages. Work out with your doctor beforehand the criteria you will use, and be in touch with your doctor the first time you decide to use a natural remedy for treating symptoms.

2: If a natural therapy does not give your child sufficient relief after a sufficient time, depending on his particular pattern, use a conventional reliever medication. Your usual reliever medication may be more effective now than before your child started the program, so administer the lowest usual dosage to start with. If you have any doubts or concerns about your child's condition, call your doctor.

WHEN TO CALL
THE DOCTOR

Be sure to work out with your doctor a mutually agreed-upon plan of action if your child experiences an asthma flare-up. You can usually treat mild flare-ups at home alone, or after a telephone consultation with your doctor. However, if symptoms persist for several days, you should call your doctor. Moderate flare-ups can also usually be handled at home, with telephone consultation; if your child does not improve significantly after you have given him the prescribed medication, again, consult your physician. **Severe flare-ups (the red zone) should always be treated at the doctor's office or emergency room.**

LEARNING TO TRUST YOURSELF

In order for this program to work, you and your child need to be comfortable with it, and that takes trust—trust in yourself and trust in the program. There's an emotional aspect and a practical aspect to establishing enough trust to reach that comfort level. If you have confidence in the practical aspects— mastering the art of administering natural therapies, knowing how to monitor, seeing the improvement in your child—you can relax emotionally. With time, you will get better and better at assuming responsibility and taking control of your child's care.

We want to reassure you that after closely observing and documenting your child's condition for some time, you will find that you have become more sensitive to subtle changes in your child. You may notice changes that are signs that his condition is worsening and a flare-up may be brewing. The more tuned in you are to early subtle changes that occur before any obvious wheezing, coughing, or shortness of breath, the better chance you have of using natural therapies effectively to prevent the flare-up. This ability is especially important when your child is too young to measure his condition with a peak flow meter. Such subtle changes include:

- mood changes—your child becomes unusually quiet, cranky, sensitive, overactive;
- breathing changes such as mouth breathing;
- complaints that he feels funny, his neck itches, yawning.

With your heightened awareness and sensitivity, you may also notice subtle positive changes after you administer the therapy, indicating that the therapy is working and you needn't worry and turn to conventional medication in a panic.

Using this program some children may become completely symptom free and not need any medication at all. Others may reduce the severity and frequency of their asthma episodes so they need reliever medication only now and then. Still others may only be able to reduce the dosages or frequency of both preventer and reliever medications. Some children respond dramatically, others take more time. But in our experience, all the children's symptoms have improved, along with their quality of life, and they have reduced the unwanted side effects of their medications by using natural therapies. Eventually, they are able to reduce their use of natural therapies as well.

However, do not become so committed to alternative treatment that you are in denial about your child's condition. Confidence that the program is working is one thing, being unable to admit when a child is in danger and needs to be seen by a physician right away is another.

It takes time, commitment, perseverance, and effort to break away from business as usual. Don't fret if it takes longer than you'd like to make progress, or if your child progresses and then relapses for a while. When relapses occur, try natural therapies, but don't delay conventional medicine too long. Don't feel that you or your child are failures if you need to use conventional drugs now and then. Remember, by taking a small dose from an inhaler early during an episode, your child can often avoid using the larger doses necessary if you allow the episode to progress.

Now that your monitoring system is in place and you and your family understand how the program works, you are ready to begin with the first crucial step: avoiding the things that trigger your child's asthma.

FIVE   AVOIDING COMMON TRIGGERS

Allergens and other asthma triggers are everywhere—they may be in the air your child breathes, the clothes she wears, the food she eats, the chair she sits in, the animals (living or stuffed) she cuddles. Fortunately, not every child is sensitive to every possible trigger, and you can significantly reduce the number and severity of asthma episodes by removing or minimizing the most offensive troublemakers at home, at school, and while traveling. That's why we feel that this is the most important and effective measure of our Natural Asthma Control Program and the place where you should begin. Once you remove as many triggers as possible, you lay a foundation for the natural therapies in the chapters to come.

The first step in avoiding triggers is to determine those you most likely need to be concerned about. If an allergist has tested your child for allergies, you will have a list of allergens to avoid. If not, take our self-assessment questionnaire to narrow down the possibilities. We recommend that you take the self-test anyway, since quite often we see patients who have been tested by allergists, but their testing failed to reveal several allergies. The next step is to make the changes in your family's life and lifestyle to reduce your child's exposure to his or her particular set of triggers. Therefore, the bulk of this chapter is devoted to how to avoid the most likely culprits affecting your child. For example, you may need to stop using scented products, to keep pets outdoors or to find a new home for them, to change your furniture and floor coverings, and to make an extra effort to reduce the risk of viral infections such as cold and flu.

Although the list of possible allergens seems daunting, bear in mind you don't necessarily need to remove them all. Just avoiding or minimizing some will reduce your child's overall toxic load, and that in turn can reduce her sensitivity to those allergens it is not possible to avoid. Just do the best you can, as did Greg's parents. In their case, it just wasn't practical to remove all of their son's triggers. For example, they could not remove the wall-to-wall carpeting because they did not own their home. But they did get a powerful new vacuum cleaner and put special anti-dust-mite covers on his bedding. And they were very committed to controlling what they could control, even if that meant stepping on other people's toes. "We are adamant about smoking," Says Karen, Greg's mother. "We don't smoke and we don't allow anybody else to smoke in the house. You need to be clear that the kid comes first, even with relatives you may be reluctant to confront because you want to keep the peace. You need to arrange or point out alternatives, and maybe be a little bit bitchy, and adopt an attitude. We just tell them, 'You can't smoke in here anymore. But we do have a front porch.'" Another child's mother says every time her family visits, "they get a little lecture."

WHAT ARE THE MOST COMMON TRIGGERS?

Although sensitivities of course vary greatly, in this chapter we cover what we have found to be the most likely triggers. Triggers fall into three basic categories:

- *Allergens* are substances that provoke an immune reaction in people who have acquired a sensitivity to them, but that are harmless in nonallergic people. Allergens are usually substances that are airborne and breathed in. According to the American Lung Association, 75 to 80 percent of children with asthma have significant allergies. Common airborne allergens include house dust, mold, pollen, and animal dander. Certain foods such as milk, fish, peanuts, eggs, wheat, and chocolate also provoke an allergic reaction in some children. The timing and pattern of symptoms offer clues as to whether your child is allergic and whether this is provoking her asthma. For example, she may sneeze and wheeze in the spring and/or the fall, when pollens are at their highest. If her symptoms stay pretty much the same year round, animals, mold, or dust may be the culprits.

• *Irritants* directly cause hypersensitive airways to constrict, without requiring the immune system to form antibodies or produce inflammatory chemicals. They affect both allergic and nonallergic children. They include air pollution, cigarette and fireplace smoke, fumes from common household supplies such as paint and cleaners, and personal products such as perfumes and hair sprays. Exercise, weather changes, infections, food additives, and certain medications including aspirin and ibuprofen can also be irritating to some children's lungs and immune systems.

• *Strong emotions* can change your child's breathing pattern, which can provoke an asthma episode; in addition, stress may worsen the underlying inflammation. These factors are discussed in Chapter 9, "Living Well with Asthma," and in Chapter 10, "Mind-Body Medicine."

ACTION STEP:

SELF-ASSESSMENT QUESTIONNAIRE

Determining what causes asthma in your child can be a complicated process. Triggers vary from child to child, and even in each child from time to time. This self assessment is based on the questionnaire we give all our asthma and allergy patients. It gives you a systematic way of ferreting out the most likely environmental triggers by making you more aware of the ones that exist in your child's life. It then gives you the opportunity to assess the effect they have on your child so you can take the most appropriate action. When completed and evaluated, it will function as a kind of "unshopping list"—a list of things you want to avoid.

To take the test:

Read down the list of potential triggers and put a check in the first column if your child is ever exposed to that trigger. In the next column, write down the frequency with which she is exposed—every day, once a week, and so on. In the final column, note the symptoms the trigger provokes and when they occur; for example, wheezing and coughing ten minutes after exposure. If your child is old enough, the two of you can work on the test together. The daily diary suggested in Chapter 4 will be an indispensable tool in filling out this questionnaire. Remember to include possible exposures outside your home—at school, a relative's or friend's house, the movie theater, restaurant or mall, a bus, train, or car. Give yourself time to fill out the questionnaire; it may take you a week or more, and you may need to review and update it periodically because children's sensitivities usually change as they grow and mature.

Assess and use the results:

You may be surprised at the number of triggers to which your child is exposed throughout the day and week. As you evaluate the questionnaire, put your initial effort into avoiding items that most obviously cause symptoms. Try to avoid them for at least two weeks and note your child's condition in the daily diary. If her symptoms improve, you know you are on the right track. Remember: if your child is allergic to pollen, during hay fever season she may be more sensitive to other allergens as well; the same holds true when she is around animals, if she is allergic to dander.

If she doesn't noticeably improve, she may have hidden or delayed reactions to other triggers. Although an allergen or trigger can cause symptoms to occur right after the initial exposure (an early phase flare-up), it can also cause another episode eight to twelve hours after the initial exposure (the late phase). This late phase is usually longer in duration than the early phase. So, the next step is to remove the things to which she is most frequently exposed, regardless of whether you notice an immediate reaction, because they are likely to be the source of delayed reactions.

It can take time to detect the myriad of triggers that are probably affecting your child. Don't get discouraged, simply continue to observe your child carefully and use the trial-and-error method to gradually clear her environment of the things that provoke her symptoms.

ACTION STEP:

AVOID ASTHMA TRIGGERS

Remember, you don't need to avoid all triggers all of the time. Simply reducing your child's exposure to those you *can* reasonably control reduces the toxic load and makes her less sensitive to others

Is your child ever exposed to:	Frequency of exposure	Symptoms
—House dust (from carpets, upholstered furniture, drapes or curtains, bedding)		
—Animal dander (from cats, dogs, birds, hamsters)		
—Stuffed animals		
—Feather pillows, comforters		
—Cockroaches		
—Mold (from damp bathroom, basement, houseplants)		
—Yeast (breads, sauces, dried fruits, cheese, mushrooms)		
—Cow's milk and dairy products (yogurt, cheese, ice cream)		
—Eggs		
—Soy foods (soy milk, tofu)		
—Wheat products (bread, crackers, cereals, pastries, pasta, pizza)		
—Smoke (from cigarettes, pipes, cigars, fireplaces, stoves, barbecues)		

Is your child ever exposed to:	Frequency of exposure	Symptoms
—Scented products (perfumes, after-shave, soaps, detergents, fabric softeners, hair products, body creams and lotions, air fresheners, scented candles)		
—Paint or solvents		
—Household products and cleaners		
—Cooking odors		
—Insecticides (moth balls, roach spray, gardening products)		
—Car, truck, bus fumes		
—Natural gas, cooking gas		
—New furnishings (carpets, furniture, plastic shower curtains)		
—Dry and/or cold air		
—Humid and/or hot air		
—Exercise		
—Colds or flu		
—Sulfites (in shrimp; frozen, canned, or dried fruits and vegetables; wine and wine vinegar; beer; fruit drinks; potato chips; baked goods; processed foods)		
—Chlorinated pools		

that you cannot avoid (remember the rain bucket?—every drop counts). For example, if your child has allergic hay fever, pollen may not provoke an episode unless she is also exposed to an irritant such as cigarette smoke.

Note: You will notice that from time to time we mention particular products that help you control triggers, for example air purifiers or bedding protectors. Please refer to the list of product suppliers in the Appendix for sources. A good all-round source is the catalog from Self-Care, which sells a laundry product that neutralizes dust mites as you launder; a spray-on product that neutralizes allergens in carpeting and upholstery; a product that reduces pet dander; air cleaners and mold reducers; high-energy-particle arresting (HEPA) filter vacuum cleaners; mite-reducing bedding, and more.

House Dust

Large quantities of house dust can act as an irritant and cause airways to narrow in defense. In small quantities dust is an allergen and causes an allergic response. The ordinary dust in your home is composed of an amazing array of substances—particles of rugs, mattresses, furniture, clothing, human skin cells, and particles of other living things, material tracked in or blown in from the outside. Most significant for asthmatics are the dust mites, animal dander, and cockroach proteins which are the primary asthma-provoking allergens.

The following tips apply to house dust in general; later on we provide special tips for these three irksome components. It is especially important to control dust in the bedroom, where your child spends at least eight hours a day. In fact, we have noticed that if asthma is worse in the morning and evening, this is a clue that dust is the culprit because getting in and out of bed stirs up dust in the mattress and bedding.

- Replace wall-to-wall carpeting with hardwood floors, ceramic tile, or linoleum. If you have carpeting, it should be tightly-woven rather than of the shag variety.
- Use throw rugs that cover less surface area and that you can wash often.
- Cover your child's mattress, box springs, and pillows with plastic or vinyl dust-proof cases; tape over the zippers and wipe down the covers once a week. If your child is also allergic to plastic fumes, use a 100-percent cotton mattress and pillow and use a cotton barrier cloth instead. Be sure to clean under the bed regularly and do not use the area for storage.
- Instead of heavy drapes, use washable curtains, aluminum or plastic blinds, or window shades.
- Avoid wall pennants in the bedroom and other decorative items that catch dust.
- Get an air purifier for as many rooms as possible. The most effective air cleaners have high-energy-particle arresting (HEPA) filters, which can trap very small particles including dust mite, animal, and cockroach proteins. We usually recommend the Alpine Air Cleaner.
- Use air filters and change your furnace filters often.
- Close and seal the heating ducts to prevent air from the furnace from entering the room. Use electric heat and, if possible, install a separate air conditioner in your child's bedroom.
- Dust often, using a damp cloth or mop—not a feather duster or broom which just pushes the dust around and throws it into the air.
- Remove stuffed upholstered furniture and replace it with wood furniture.
- Wash your child's stuffed animals frequently and don't let your child sleep with them.

- Wash sheets weekly in hot water.
- Clean regularly, using nontoxic cleaning materials.
- If you vacuum, do so while your child is out of the house, and use a vacuum with a HEPA filter.

Dust Mites

This is probably the most potent allergen in house dust. These tiny creatures are related to spiders and ticks and live on specks of dust. Invisible to the naked eye, they are everywhere you find dust—especially bedding, upholstered furniture, carpeting, drapery, and stuffed animals, to name the most obvious. Mites, though no fun to think about, are not harmful to people who are not allergic. And the mites themselves are not the problem—it's the protein in their droppings, which they leave everywhere. The number of mites has increased tremendously because we now live in much "tighter" houses to save energy. The reduced ventilation and increased warmth help mites flourish.

All the tips for reducing house dust will also reduce mites. However, if it is too costly to replace flooring and furnishings, you may try treating materials with a special spray containing tannic acid. This compound found in coffee, tea, and cocoa may neutralize the protein that is responsible for allergic reactions. Some experts recommend you also use benzyl benzoate, a chemical that kills mites, but a less toxic solution, and one that we recommend, is to simply keep the room well-humidified so the dust doesn't fly around.

Animal Dander

The problem is a protein in their dander—flakes of skin—and in their saliva, not in their fur or feathers. However, when animals clean themselves, the allergen in their saliva attaches to their hair or feathers, and thus hair or feathers can indirectly cause an allergic reaction. Animal allergens are found on the animals themselves, of course, but they also accumulate in carpeting, furniture upholstery, and bedding. Allergens also become airborne as they dry; as they float through the air your child may breath them in, and they can even stick to walls, clothing, and other surfaces around the home. To keep allergic reactions to pets to a minimum, follow the same housekeeping and furnishing procedures as for house dust and dust mites. Bear in mind that it takes up to six weeks of repeated and thorough cleaning to completely clean dander from a home. In addition:

- If you don't own a pet, don't get one unless it is a dander-free animal such as a fish or turtle.
- Keep furred and feathered pets such as cats, dogs, and birds outside as much as possible. Build a shelter for them to soften the blow to your child and make the animals more comfortable.
- If you can't keep them outdoors, keep them away from carpeted areas and out of your child's bedroom.
- If your child still reacts to dander, consider finding the pets another home (see box, "Saying Goodbye to Fluffy," on page 84).
- Give cats and dogs a bath once a week to reduce the amount of allergens they produce; also brush cats and dogs regularly so they don't feel the need to groom themselves frequently and spread allergens in their saliva.
- Clean pet areas frequently with nontoxic cleaners.
- Don't use bedding containing feathers or down.
- Avoid visits to friends or relatives with allergenic pets.

SAYING GOODBYE TO FLUFFY

Finding a new home for a beloved pet can be emotionally devastating for your child and for the whole family. Here are some ways to ease the blow.

- Be honest—state clearly that the reason the pet must go is because it is making the child's allergies and asthma worse; let your child know that you have decided that the family must say goodbye so that he or she will feel better. Do not blame the change on the pet's behavior or say that Fluffy will be happier somewhere else.

- Do not use the term "getting rid of."

- Talk about it among the family. Ask your child and his siblings how they feel about living without the animal. Don't let siblings cast blame on you or their allergic brother or sister. Recognize that there may be anger at you or that the child may blame himself. Recognize that there will be a grieving process for the loss of a pet— counteract this by encouraging the family to talk about the fun they had and the love they felt, and let them know that these memories will never be lost.

- Get everyone involved in finding the pet a new home— your veterinarian will be a good resource. Make sure your child approves of the new owners and sees that the pet is in a good home. If he or she does not approve, ask why.

- If the loss still seems too traumatic, consider redoubling your efforts to remove other allergens and triggers from your child's environment; exposure to these added troublemakers can aggravate pet allergies, and removal of other triggers may make pet allergens more tolerable.

Cockroaches

Recent studies show that cockroaches, already an unpopular species, are a potent allergen and trigger of asthma. According to Patricia Robuck of Johns Hopkins School of Public Health, asthma sufferers who are allergic to roaches and who are continually exposed to them appear to have much more serious asthma than other asthmatics—they need more medication, are hospitalized more and die more frequently from asthma. This finding is especially troublesome for city kids, who are the most exposed to roaches. It is estimated that about 50 percent of children with asthma in large cities such as New York City are allergic to roaches.

According to Robuck, all neighborhoods in large cities that have a warm, humid season have cockroaches. That means that swanky apartment buildings have as much potential for harboring roaches as do poorer neighborhoods—they just exterminate more effectively. The allergens from roaches are primarily found in their saliva, but also in their feces, egg casings, and the outside of their bodies. That means wherever a cockroach has walked, it may leave behind allergens. In a Johns Hopkins study that sampled dust in homes where people said they had never seen roaches, researchers said they often found cockroach allergen. The major source was the kitchen and bathroom, but the allergen can get tracked throughout the home. A study published in a 1998 issue of *The Journal of Allergy and Clinical Immunology* suggests that removing cockroach allergens from the bedroom may be particularly important, possibly because children spend so much time there.

Getting rid of roaches is difficult, as any big-city dweller knows, especially if you live in an apartment building. That's because you must get neighbors to act too, or else the roaches will just recolonize your place again when the pesticide wears off. But it's not hopeless:

- Don't leave dirty dishes, crumbs, pet food, or puddles of water overnight. Store food in tight containers.

- Some cockroaches are especially fond of beer, so rinse all beer containers before storing for recycling, and wipe up any spills.

- Remove hiding places—store papers, cartons, empty bottles, and other recyclables outside. Be especially wary of bags and cardboard boxes you bring from outside the home.

- Repair leaky faucets to remove sources of moisture. Repair all areas where roaches could enter—cracks, gaps, and holes in walls and floors; caulk around pipes.

- Clean all surfaces thoroughly with soap and water; a damp rag or a quick dusting won't help.

- Use the least toxic insecticide you can find. We recommend boric acid because it is nonallergenic and a relatively safe treatment. Sprinkle it wherever you see roaches, but avoid areas where children or pets can reach it because swallowing it or allowing it to come into contact with eyes or skin can be harmful. Less toxic still are home-made mixtures of either equal parts oatmeal or flour with plaster of paris, or equal parts of baking soda and sugar; spread this around the infested area.

- If you use an insect spray, try to find products that are nontoxic to humans and use only if your child is outside the house because your child may have a reaction to the pesticide. Professional extermination is most effective, but if you do it yourself, "bombs," which disperse a fine aerosol mist, are the most successful. Be sure to follow directions exactly. Roach traps, although less effective than sprays and powders, are nontoxic to children.

Mold or Mildew

Mold (also called mildew) forms on fallen leaves, soil, debris, and other moist surfaces. It thrives in damp basements, closets, window moldings, bathrooms, air conditioners and humidifiers, and houseplants. Most homes outside the dry Southwest are moist enough to grow molds, which reproduce by releasing tiny spores into the air. Many of our patients are from upstate New York, where mold and mildew are a year-round problem. We find that if our patients take these measures their allergies improve significantly and they become less allergic to other allergens as well because they have taken a major load off their systems.

Mold spores can cause allergies year-round, but this allergen is most bothersome from spring to late fall. Some experts theorize that molds are such potent asthma provokers because their smaller size allows them to penetrate the lungs more deeply than pollen. Another theory is that they interact synergistically with other allergens. To reduce mold in your home:

- Clean damp, mold-prone areas regularly (shower stalls and drains, sinks, refrigerators, garbage pail, basements, shower curtains, bathroom tile, behind the toilet, window moldings). Use borax and vinegar mixed with water in a spray bottle; spray on and wipe off the mold. A commercial mold remover that is also nontoxic is AMF Safety Clean; AMF 158 Mildew Control is more potent. Both are available at hardware stores. Clorox bleach (1 cup per 10 cups water) is also a potent mold killer, but bleach is toxic to the environment, so use sparingly.

- Keep your bathroom unfriendly to mold by keeping the air dry and circulating with an exhaust fan; this lets surfaces, towels, and washcloths dry quickly. Avoid leaving damp clothing and towels in the hamper. Wash your shower curtain periodically in hot water with detergent and bleach.

- Change pillows at least every year because old, sweaty pillows can be incubators for molds.

- Use an air purifier.

- Look for mold under carpets and rugs and behind loose wallpaper and wall paneling. Use washable cotton or wool throw rugs instead of large rugs or wall-to-wall carpeting.

- Dry out your basement if it is damp; ventilate it and keep a light burning to discourage mold.

- Place a piece of charcoal in bookcases; this helps absorb dampness and prevents books from getting musty.

- Check with your health care provider about air conditioners and dehumidifiers and use them knowledgeably. The ideal humidity for asthmatics is between 25 and 40 percent because this allows the mucus membranes and hair-like cilia to keep the airways clean. Anything higher than that can irritate lungs and encourage the growth of mold and mites in the home. Bear in mind that if used incorrectly, air conditioners and dehumidifiers can actually encourage mold growth, so keep them clean and disinfected using nontoxic cleansers.

- Clean your child's nebulizer, inhaler, and spacer regularly.

- Keep the mold in houseplants from releasing their spores into the air by placing a layer of gravel on top of the soil. Don't overwater them or let water accumulate and stand in their saucers. Repot plants outdoors away from your asthmatic child to avoid releasing spores into the air. Give plants away or keep them outdoors if they continue to trigger your child's asthma. Watch out for dried plants, too, because they often harbor mold.

- Replace your evergreen Christmas tree with an artificial tree. Real trees may cause mold allergy to flare-up.

- Keep the compost bin or pile as far from home as possible.

- Don't accumulate old newspapers and magazines.

- Consider moving shrubs away from the house or pruning them severely to let in more air and light. If your home is in a shady area or near a stream, it is more prone to mold.

- Limit your child's play or chores that involve leaves, lawns, and hay. If he does chores such as sweeping, gardening, or raking leaves, have him wear a face mask to protect him from allergens and irritants.

Pollen

Pollen consists of minuscule particles that carry the plant's male genetic material to a female plant. The particles travel through the air and are invisible to the naked eye until they settle and accumulate as a fine yellow powdery blanket that covers cars, mailboxes, and other outdoor objects in the spring and summer. Pollen from trees, weeds, and grasses is responsible for most hay fever—flower pollen allergies are rare because the pollen is heavier and is usually carried by insects, not the wind. Some pollen is so light it is carried as far as four hundred miles out to sea and two miles high into the air.

Try to avoid exposing your child to pollen as much as possible. Determine whether your child is allergic to tree, grass, or weed pollen and then find out when that type of pollen peaks in your region. This tells you when you need to be especially vigilant. You can get your local pollen and mold counts by calling 1-800-9-POLLEN, or visit www.aaaai.org/patpub/nab/index.html or www.allergy-info.com for more information. To reduce your child's exposure to pollens:

- Keep your child inside as much as possible when pollen counts are highest; this usually occurs during the early morning hours, between 5:00 A.M. and 10:00 A.M. Pollen counts drop in the midafternoon.

- Use an air purifier. Use an air conditioner instead of opening windows in your home and car.

- Don't hang bedding or clothes outside to dry because they can collect pollen.

- Try to get your child to change clothes and shower away the pollen after being outdoors. At least have him wash his hands and face. Pollen collects on clothes, hair, face, hands, and body. So unless he removes the pollen, your child keeps breathing it in and transfers it to his pillows at night.

- If you live near the ocean, go to the seashore as often and as long as possible to give your child pollen-free air.

Food Allergens

Food is a common but often unrecognized asthma trigger in children. According to the American Lung Association, 6 percent of children under the age of two have food allergies, and 1 to 2 percent of children over age ten have food allergies. The American Medical Association reports that 8 percent of children under the age of six experience food intolerances. In our practice we have found these percentages to be much higher—in fact, *most* of the

PLANT A "SNEEZELESS" GARDEN

It's difficult to control your child's exposure to pollen, but one place you can control is right your own backyard. According to the American Lung Association the following plants are *least* likely to cause allergic reactions. So if you have a garden and a child who is allergic to pollen, *emphasize:*

- TREES: Chinese tallow, tulip tree, silk tree, strawberry tree, catalpa, pine, pear, podocarpus, dogwood, fir, palm, redwood, fig, mulberry, jacaranda, plum, crape myrtle, silk oak, coral tree, orchid tree, redbud, maidenhair, magnolia, chorisia.
- SHRUBS: nandina, oleander, yucca, manzanita, pyracantha, viburnum, grevillea, pittosporum, hibiscus, boxwood, verbena, cinquefoil, tradescantia, sedum.
- GRASSES: dichondra, rye, blue, fescue, irish moss, hippocrepis comosa, mazus reptans.
- FLOWERS: poppy, azalea, camellia, bougainvillea, solanum, cymbidium, begonia, pansy, tulip, ranunculus, iris, daffodil, peony.

The following plants are *most* likely to cause allergic reactions and should be *avoided* in your plantings:

- TREES: olive, ash, sycamore, sweetgum, acacia, elm, walnut, privet, alder, oak, pecan, birch, almond, fruitless mulberry, cottonwood, poplar, willow.
- PLANTS: juniper, elderberry, thuja, privet, rhamnus, ceanothus.
- GRASSES: Bermuda.
- FLOWERS: amaranthus, ceanothus.

children we treat are sensitive to foods. They either have allergies, which involve a specific mechanism in which measurable amounts of the immunoglobulin E and/or G are released, or sensitivities, in which we cannot measure the biochemicals responsible for the reaction. While there are tests to detect allergies, there are no reliable tests yet for detecting sensitivities—only observation gives us clues. In our practice, we seldom distinguish between allergies and sensitivities because it doesn't matter which mechanism is at play: avoidance of the offending substance is still the main treatment.

We find that the foods that most often provoke asthma symptoms are milk, eggs, soy, and wheat products. Often when we eliminate these foods from the diet, the immune system calms down enough so that asthmatic children do not have a strong reaction to other triggers including animal dander, pollens, and house dust. If the daily diary suggests that your child may have food allergies or sensitivities to these or other foods, refer to Chapter 6, "Food as Healer."

Airborne Irritants

Even if your child is not allergic, you need to be vigilant about irritating gases and particles that cause bronchoconstriction. You'll run across irritants both indoors and out, but recent evidence suggests indoor air may contain more irritants than outdoor air.

- An estimated two hundred thousand to one million asthmatic children have their condition worsened by cigarette smoke, according to the American Lung Association. Don't smoke, and make it a rule that no one smokes in your home or car. Patronize only nonsmoking restaurants and/or sit in nonsmoking sections. Ask for nonsmoking rental cars and motel rooms.

- Fireplaces and wood burning stoves are a source of airborne irritants and allergens. Your child needs to sit well away from their smoke and fumes. Better still, keep him out of rooms with wood fires.

- Avoid scented products, such as candles, room deodorizers and fresheners, laundry soaps, bath soaps, and fabric softeners.

- Avoid wearing perfumes and scented body care products such as lotions, deodorants, and hair products.

- Avoid other strongly scented products such as paint, solvents, and strong household cleaning products.

- Avoid using aerosol products of any kind around your child because they put tiny particles in the air that can linger and cause irritation. Powder or talc can also put fine particles in the air that act as irritants.

- Use an exhaust fan when you cook to keep the air moving and irritant-free.

- Replace all harsh cleaning and household products with nontoxic products.

- Avoid soft plastics and plastic wrap for food; use cellophane or waxed paper instead, and wood, ceramic, glass, or steel bowls and containers for serving and storage.

- Avoid insecticides in the home and garden, including mothballs.

Avoid as many other irritating chemicals as possible. This is especially important if your child is allergic or sensitive to them because they can create inflammation, but we advise everyone to avoid them because they increase the toxic load. These include: gasoline; diesel fuel; natural gas; marking pen; dry cleaning chemicals; paints; solvents; varnish and shellac; synthetic fabrics such as dacron, polyester, orlon, and acrylic; plastic shower curtains; new carpeting, carpet backing, and carpet glue; and furniture made of particle board, which contains formaldehyde.

Activity and Exercise

Exercise is almost guaranteed to spark asthma symptoms, and until all too recently, it was thought that children with asthma needed to "sit it out." The stereotype was of the pale and thin (or pudgy) child, only able to watch from the sidelines. But exercise is so beneficial for your child that it pays to learn how to encourage, rather than discourage, your child from enjoying physical activity. (See box, "The Good Trigger"). When your child's asthma is under

THE GOOD TRIGGER

The many well-documented benefits of regular exercise are no less true for asthmatics than nonasthmatic children. In the first place, an active childhood sets a pattern for an active adulthood and decreased risk of cardiovascular problems, diabetes, obesity, osteoporosis, and several types of cancer. Exercise is a superb stress reliever and natural outlet for your child's inherent exuberance, for any feelings of aggressiveness, competitiveness, and need to strive for accomplishment. This is particularly useful for the child with asthma who may feel stress and doubts about self-worth more keenly than other children. Children with asthma also benefit from physical activity because it can strengthen lungs and maintain good general health and conditioning. As a result, your child experiences less shortness of breath during exercise and can better handle toxic substances and clear them from the body.

Evidence that exercise does reduce symptoms overall comes, for example, from an Australian study which involved children with mild to severe asthma. The children worked out with professional swim coaches for five months; at the end of the program, they were swimming vigorously for one hour five times a week. When they were evaluated, the children had all gained weight but had decreased body fat. Their symptoms were reduced and they used less medication. In this case, a potential trigger is actually a natural therapy.

control, your child should be able to run and play and even compete in sports just as other children do. Many famous athletes have asthma, but this did not stop them from achieving great things, even competing in the Olympics. Consider, for example, 1996 gold medal swimmers Tom Dolan and Amy Van Dyken, champion diver Greg Louganis, and track and field star Jackie Joyner-Kersee.

It helps if you understand how exercise can act as trigger. Strenuous, continuous exercise causes your child to breathe rapidly through his mouth. Thus, the air that reaches his airways has not had a chance to be warmed and humidified by the nose and upper airways. This sudden exposure to colder, drier air can cause the airways to become twitchier and the muscles surrounding them to go into spasm. In exercise-induced asthma, the symptoms generally subside without any medication within a few minutes, but they may persist up to an hour.

We cannot overemphasize the positive role exercise should play in your child's asthma control program. Even though it can sometimes act as a trigger, do not make the mistake of discouraging your child from physical activity or allowing him to become a couch potato. However, if your child is out of shape now because of a reluctance or inability to be physically active in the past, he may be embarrassed to start participating now. Therefore, be extra gentle and reassuring if this is the case. To get the ball rolling, join your child in activities and games you both like and are capable of doing. Walk, play catch or Frisbee, take a leisurely bike ride. Encourage your other children, if any, to do this also. By beginning in the safety of a family environment, your child will feel more self confident when he is at school and out with his playmates.

To reduce the chance that exercise will provoke asthma, follow these tips:

- Consider the level of other triggers your child is exposed to during exercise. Are pollen counts high? Is the air pollution bad? If so, your child may need to modify physical activity. Conversely, if you can minimize exposure to these factors, your child will be less sensitive to exercise.

- Teach your child to warm up gradually at the start of a strenuous activity. He should start slowly and gradually increase the intensity of activity. In addition, make sure he is properly conditioned for the sport.

- Choose exercise wisely. Try to find an activity that your child likes and is comfortable with. Treadmill tests have shown that asthma symptoms are usually triggered within six to eight minutes of beginning a strenuous activity, such as running, which leads to rapid mouth breathing. So sports which require only short intermittent bursts of intense activity may be best for your child, at least until his asthma is under better control. These include baseball, football, volleyball, wrestling, weight lifting, golf, tennis, swimming, gymnastics, and short-distance track and field events, rather than long-distance running, cross-country skiing, soccer, cycling, or aerobic dance.

- Consider the conditions in which your child exercises. Children are often steered toward swimming because it takes place in warm humid air. However, breathing in air with chlorine fumes could act as a trigger in some sensitive children, and the mold and mites found in this environment could be triggers in some children. We advise that you give your child extra antioxidant supplements before he goes swimming. In addition, you may want to limit, modify, or avoid activities during cold weather or that are enjoyed in cold environments such as skiing, ice hockey, or ice skating.

- Have your child wear a scarf around his nose and mouth when he plays or exercises in cold weather. This creates a pocket of warmed, humidified air which your child can breath in again. This technique is even more effective if you put a surgeon's mask under the scarf; alternatively you could buy a cold-air mask, available at pharmacies. If possible, remind your child to try to breathe through his nose rather than his mouth to better warm and humidify the air.

- Be aware that your child may need to take medication before playing a sport or game or running a race. As you progress through the steps of our Natural Asthma Control Program, you may find this is no longer necessary. Or you may discover a natural therapy that works as well as conventional drugs to prevent an exercise-induced episode.

- Be sure to talk to your child's coach and physical education teacher about asthma and exercise.

Weather

Weather can trigger asthma. For example, tests have shown that cold air provokes flare-ups in most children who have the condition. Dry air is also a provocative agent. In some children, rainy days are risky. Therefore, be on the lookout for sudden weather changes; depending on the weather conditions that affect your child, you may want to:

- Limit the amount of time your child plays outdoors during cold, dry weather, and to use a scarf or ski mask to cover your child's mouth and nose in very cold weather.

- Pay attention to weather changes, which affect airborne allergens, and take extra precautions. For example, wind scatters more of them through the air; heavy rain washes the air clean, but dampness may increase mold; a thermal inversion may increase the concentration of air pollution. Studies have shown that the number of asthma patients requiring emergency care rises dramatically after thunderstorms.

Colds, Flu, and Other Infectious Illnesses

Viral upper respiratory infections are perhaps the most common trigger of asthma symptoms in young children. When a virus infects the sinuses, nose, throat, airways, or lungs, a number of reactions occur. Certain cells in the airways release inflammatory chemicals such as *histamine* and *leukotrienes*. These chemicals cause swelling of the airways and an increase in mucus secretion; they may also cause bronchoconstriction. As a result, the airways narrow and asthma symptoms occur. Nighttime asthma flare-ups can be due in part to excess mucus of sinusitis or post-nasal drip, chronic conditions found in 70 percent of asthmatics. In addition, certain childhood respiratory infections increase the likelihood that a child will develop asthma later on; these include bronchiolitis, bronchitis, croup, and pneumonia.

The tips that follow will help you reduce your child's risk of becoming infected. In later chapters we explain how to prevent and treat infection using natural therapies such as nutritional supplements and herbs.

- Remind your child to wash her hands often.

- Make sure your child's immune system is strong so she can better resist viral and bacterial infections. Feed her a healthy diet (Chapter 6), give her nutritional supple ments (Chapter 7), give her an immune-boosting herbal tonic (Chapter 8), and help her cope with stressful emotions (Chapter 10).

- If your doctor recommends it, consider taking your child for a flu shot. However, we generally advise parents against flu shots because they can compromise the immune system.

- Use natural therapies such as herbs to treat colds and flu, and avoid giving your child antibiotics.

- Within reason, try to avoid exposing your child to viruses if she gets severe asthma flare-ups; for example, keep her away from adults and children who have colds and flu. If your child goes to school, it's impossible to avoid exposure, so give her extra immune-enhancing herbs and nutrients such as echinacea and vitamin C.

Medications

In some children, aspirin and other anti-inflammatory medications such as ibuprofen can trigger asthma symptoms. It is wise to avoid them and any products containing them (read labels carefully); these include cold tablets, antihistamine and cold combination pills, medication for menstrual symptoms, and a variety of prescription drugs. Tylenol, the common medication given to children, is not a known asthma trigger.

This chapter has been about the "don'ts" because avoiding common triggers is a giant step in controlling your child's asthma. But you can't avoid all the potential factors, so you also need to take other positive steps to alleviate the underlying inflammation and reduce his or her sensitivity, and alleviate symptoms when they occur. The following chapter will show you how to use food to do just that.

SIX

FOOD AS HEALER

After avoiding triggers, we have found that making sure a child eats a healthy diet is the next most crucial step in our Natural Asthma Control Program. Food affects all of your child's systems, twenty-four hours a day. It can help heal or it can hurt your child because the right kind of food supplies the building blocks and energy your child needs to grow up healthy and strong and to keep her immune and respiratory systems functioning optimally.

But if you're like most parents, you lead a busy, complicated life and are happy to get *any* food into your child, let alone feed her the perfect diet. The temptation to just kick back and eat junk food is everywhere. There are so many food choices. Children are notoriously finicky when it comes to eating, and the dinner table can become a battleground even in homes where asthma is not an issue. Not to mention that feeding kids with asthma can be even more of a challenge because so many have food allergies and sensitivities, making food selection more complicated. Yet it's doubly important.

Clearly, you have your work cut out for you. In this chapter, we aim to help. We explain how what your child eats and drinks can either improve your child's asthma or worsen it. We provide you with specific action steps to help you assess your child's current diet, adopt new eating patterns to more closely approximate an optimum diet, and avoid foods to which your child is allergic. And we include tried-and-true tricks of the trade for getting wholesome, healing foods into a wary, resistant child. Because prevention is so much easier than treatment, we include a special section on how to avoid causing allergies and asthma to develop in your younger children and infants. Finally, we provide guidelines to determine whether you should take your child to a professional nutritionist, how to find a good one, and what to expect in the way of treatment.

This chapter helps you find a way to feed your child a cleaner, purer, more nourishing diet. By gradually adopting our suggestions, you will provide a diet that lessens your child's exposure to toxins, helps the liver and other systems detoxify the harmful substances already accumulated in his body, and strengthens his ability to handle unavoidable toxins such as pollution and any asthma medications he is taking. In the process, your child's asthma will improve, and you will also lower his risk of infection, allergies and—as a bonus—a host of other serious conditions from heart disease to diabetes to cancer.

> **REMINDER:** When you take any of the steps in this chapter, remember to continue your child's regular medical treatment. Do not reduce asthma medications on your own—do this only under the advice and supervision of your child's physician. If your child shows any of the danger signs of an asthma flare-up (see page 59, Chapter 4), seek medical attention immediately.

WHAT'S WRONG WITH THE STANDARD AMERICAN DIET?

It's no coincidence that the abbreviation for Standard American Diet is "SAD." Numerous surveys show that our intake of certain nutrients is shockingly inadequate, while our intake of others is way too high. We are overfed but undernourished—it's no wonder that as a nation, we are getting fatter and sicker every year, and so are our children.

Simply put, the average child's diet is too low in healthful vitamins, minerals, and fiber; too high in refined starches and sugars; and contains an imbalance of fats. Take, for example, the RDAs (Recommended Dietary Allowances) established by the U.S. government, which define the levels of the essential vitamins and minerals adequate to prevent deficiency diseases. According to a recent U.S. Department of Agriculture survey, which studied the three-day food intake of 21,500 people, **not one single person** consumed 100 percent of the RDA for the ten nutrients included in the survey. This is *really sad*, because in our view, the RDAs are the absolute *minimum* anyone should be getting.

What's true for adults is true for our children. A number of surveys over the past five years have shown that children don't eat enough fruits and vegetables, and that they fall short on many vitamins and minerals. A survey recently conducted by the American Medical Association found that while parents believe they have a good understanding of a balanced diet, they aren't making use of that knowledge. For example, 72 percent of the parents were unconcerned about the amount of soft drinks and junk food consumed by their children. These are "empty" foods, devoid of nutrition, and leave very little room in kids' tummies for healthful foods. As the parent of an asthmatic child, you simply cannot afford to be in that 72 percent.

Eating the standard American diet fails to supply the nutrients needed for cell growth and regeneration, including the lungs and entire respiratory system. It places a high burden on your child's immune system and detoxifying systems, and creates more inflammation and hypersensitivity. What's more, it includes many foods such as milk, wheat, eggs, and artificial food additives that are responsible for the majority of the food allergies that help provoke asthma flare-ups. Along with a sedentary lifestyle, the standard American diet leads to obesity. Today, about one in five American children are considered to be overweight. Being overweight worsens asthma symptoms. Not to mention that overweight children often have a poor self-image and express feelings of inferiority and rejection. They are often teased, left out of other children's games, and become less active and more isolated in a vicious circle of toxic emotions.

WHAT SHOULD YOUR CHILD BE EATING?

The following optimum daily eating plan gives you a general idea of the food groups and the amount of each to aim for each day. Similar to the USDA Food Guide Pyramid, it is high in nutrients, reduces the toxic burden, and helps eliminate toxins. As is the case with avoiding triggers, this diet is a *preventer* of chronic asthma, rather than a *reliever* of acute symptoms. Eating this way helps strengthen your child's body, including the lungs, supports normal immune function, reduces mucus formation, minimizes bronchial spasms, and calms inflammation. This helps prevent asthma as well as the colds, flu, and allergies that can provoke asthma symptoms.

Although we continue to fine-tune our recommendations based on the latest research, we have been prescribing this way of eating for many years. We have gotten remarkable results when parents make appropriate changes in their child's diet a cornerstone in their Natural Asthma Control Program. Our eating plan is vegetarian or near vegetarian. It emphasizes plant foods and consists mainly of vegetables, fruits, grains and beans. It plays down animal products such as cow's milk and meat because these foods are associated with a slew of serious diseases and conditions, including several types of cancer, heart disease, osteoporosis, and asthma. Plant foods, on the other hand, help promote better health (see box, "The Power of Plants," page 111). However, again we urge moderation. Although plants can be powerfully healing, veganism (a form of vegetarianism that excludes not only the flesh of animals, but also any animal products such as dairy products, eggs, and honey) may be too extreme for most children. This is because although it is high in many nutrients, an all-plant diet takes a lot of planning to ensure children are supplied with enough other nutrients that are readily available in animal foods, such as calcium, zinc, and vitamins D and B–12.

Optimum Diet

We generally recommend the following amounts for children aged 6–12 and who are 45" to 57" tall. For other children, use the same number of servings, but adjust the serving size up or down as follows: For children aged 12 and up and 57" tall or more, at least double the portion size (especially if undergoing a growth spurt). For children aged 2–6 and from 34" to 45" in height, cut the portions roughly in half. For children ages 1–2, give 1 tablespoon per year of life if you are giving solid food.

1. Low-starch vegetables

Number of servings: 3 to 4 per day

Size of serving: 1 cup (measured uncooked)

Broccoli, carrots, spinach, lettuce, onions, celery, string beans, summer squash, endive, cabbage, cucumbers, asparagus, chard, peppers, parsley, rhubarb, sprouts, tomatoes. Include one 1-cup serving (measured un-cooked) of high-calcium leafy greens such as spinach, beet greens, collards, kale, dandelion and turnip greens, or bok choy.

2. *Starchy vegetables*

Number of servings: 1 per day

Size of serving: $1/2$–1 cup (measured cooked)

Potatoes, yams, sweet potatoes, parsnips, beets, winter squash, turnips, artichokes, taro, jerusalem artichokes.

3. *Whole grains*

Number of servings: 4 per day

Size of serving: $1/2$ cup cooked grains; add 1–2 slices of whole grain bread, if desired

Brown rice, oats, corn, millet, barley, buckwheat, amaranth, quinoa, wheat (couscous, bulgar, wheat berries, whole wheat cooked cereal), triticale, rye.

4. *Fresh fruit*

Number of servings: 2–4 per day

Size of serving: 1 fruit, or $1/2$ cup

Apples, apricots, berries, banana, cantaloupe or other melon in season, cherries, peaches, plums, oranges, grapefruit, grapes, kiwi. The more colorful and the deeper the color the better; choose one orange-colored fruit per day.

5. *Beans*

Number of servings: if primary source of protein, 4 servings per day; if not, 1 serving

Size of serving: $1/2$ cup cooked

Split peas, lentils, kidney beans, navy beans, chickpeas,

aduki beans, black beans, white beans, mung or soy beans, tofu.

6. Meat, fish, poultry

Number of servings: if included, limit to 1 serving every other day

Size of serving: 4–5 ounces

Cold-water fish such as tuna, salmon, mackerel, and herring are preferable; fresh lean meats such as organically raised free-range turkey or chicken in moderation. Eggs should be organic, free-range, local, and fresh; limit to 3–4 per week if you open the yolk during cooking; more if using the white only, or if cooking without opening the yolk, such as poaching or soft-boiling. (Cooking an open yolk makes the cholesterol it contains more harmful.)

7. Milk (dairy or nondairy)

Number of servings: up to 3 per day

Size of serving: 1 cup low-fat milk, or 1 ounce cheese

Vegetable milks such as soy, rice, almond, or oat milk and milk products are preferable to animal milks such as cow and goat, with the possible exception of $3/4$ cup of organic yogurt. Look for vegetable milks that are fortified with calcium and other nutrients normally present in cow's milk.

8. Essential fats

Two to three teaspoons of unrefined vegetable oils of flax, canola, or sesame seed. Use only organic, expeller-pressed oils, and keep all oils refrigerated once opened. Do not heat or cook with these oils; use them in salad and vegetable dressings; stir into soups, stews, and cooked grains and cereals just before serving; add to shakes or smoothies.

9. *Other oils*

Small amounts of olive oil and canola oil for cooking and dressings.

10. *Nuts and seeds*

A small amount of fresh, unsalted nuts and seeds (2 to 4 tablespoons) per day or nut butter if desired. Home roasted sunflower, sesame, or pumpkin seeds are a delicious snack or garnish.

11. *Booster herbs and spices*

Garlic, onions, ginger, and shiitake mushrooms as part of cooked dishes, soups, and teas.

12. *Water*

Aim for six to eight 8-ounce glasses per day—purified or spring water is preferred. To find out how your water measures up in terms of contaminants, call the EPA hotline (800-426-4791) to find a certified testing laboratory near you.

13. *Processed or convenience foods*

Little or none; if you must, save for special occasions such as parties: candy, cookies, pastries, muffins, pies, sugary sodas and drinks; ice cream; potato chips and other fried snack foods; commercial cereals; fatty fast foods such as fries and burgers; foods containing hydrogenated oils.

Why Is This Optimum?

Our diet is better for your child than the standard American diet because:

Our diet emphasizes whole fresh foods that are high in essential vitamins, minerals, and other nutrients. Many vitamins and minerals have been associated with normal immune system function and a lessening of asthma symptoms, particularly vitamin C, vitamin E, vitamin B-6, and the minerals selenium and zinc. Vitamin A (and its precursor, beta-carotene) is needed to maintain healthy lungs. Magnesium is needed for normal muscle function to avoid bronchospasm. Low levels of selenium and vitamins C and E in the diet are associated with increased risk of asthma.

Our diet is moderate in protein. Children need to eat enough protein because it is used to repair and replace cells and is the building block for biochemicals such as enzymes and brain chemicals. The healthiest sources are beans, lentils, nuts (high in vitamins, minerals, and fiber) and cold-water fish (high in omega-3 essential fatty acids). The protein in the standard American diet is often too high, which strains your child's body, depletes it of calcium, and creates toxins; furthermore, in the standard American diet most of the protein comes from animal products, which have been associated with serious diseases.

Our diet has balanced amounts of healthy fats. Children need healthy fats in order to grow and develop properly. Monounsaturated fats and essential fatty acids appear to be the most healthful. Monounsaturated fats neither raise cholesterol nor become easily oxidized in the body (see Free Radicals in Chapter 1). Essential fatty acids (EFAs) come in two main forms: omega-6 and omega-3. The typical American diet has an excess of omega-6 (found in meats and many popular vegetable oils such as corn and safflower), which is associated with the production of inflammatory chemicals in the body. Omega-3 fatty acids balance or counteract that tendency to cause inflammation—an attribute that is particularly important for children with asthma. The standard American diet contains imbalances in EFAs which are associated with eczema and allergic reactions as well as asthma. The best sources of omega-3 fatty acids are cold water fish, flax seed (and flax seed oil), and walnuts. A 1996 Australian study found that half of the children who were prone to asthma and who ate fresh fish such as salmon, tuna, and mackerel at least once a week avoided asthma symptoms.

Our diet is high in unrefined carbohydrates and fiber. Carbohydrates are needed to fuel the body and create energy. Complex carbohydrates are found in whole grains, beans, nuts, fruits, and starchy vegetables. Such starchy foods are generally relatively high in vitamins and minerals. They also contain more fiber than simple sugars and refined carbohydrates such as white bread. Fiber is needed to maintain healthy bowel function in order to eliminate toxins from the body; your child should have at least one bowel movement per day. By way of contrast, the standard American diet is low in complex carbohydrates and favors refined, simple carbohydrates.

Our diet minimizes highly processed foods. Convenience and processed foods are made of refined carbohydrates (white flour and sugar) and unhealthy fats that can hurt a child with asthma in many ways. They have had their nutrients stripped away and supply mostly empty calories; in trying to digest and metabolize them, your body actually uses more energy and nutrients than the refined carbohydrate can provide. Sugar—even sugar in fruit juice—impairs the immune system for up to five hours after it is eaten. Sugars also contribute to "leaky gut syndrome." This condition compromises the lining of your child's intestines, making it more permeable. As a result, your child absorbs more antigens and toxic substances, overtaxing the liver and triggering an immune reaction that results in asthma flare-ups. Refined carbohydrates may cause intestinal gas or reflux, which puts pressure on the diaphragm and worsens asthma symptoms. They stress the adrenal glands, which can lead to the production of chemicals that cause inflammation and bronchoconstriction. Highly processed foods cause the body to use up or lose important nutrients such as vitamins A and C, magnesium, selenium, calcium, and omega–3 fatty acids. And finally, they are full of additives such as food colorings, artificial flavors, preservatives, and pesticides, which can cause allergic reactions and add to the toxic burden.

Our diet emphasizes water as the main beverage. Water makes up half of your child's body weight and supports all the body's processes; it collects wastes and toxins and carries them to the organs of elimination and is needed to soften the body's waste so it can be easily eliminated. Plain water is a much healthier drink than sugar-laden fruit juices and sodas. Sodas also contain phosphates which deplete the body of calcium. However, we do not recommend tap water in most cases. We recommend bottled or filtered water because of the increasing danger that drinking water may contain dangerous pollutants. Each year, more than forty-six million people drink water that fails to meet Environmental Protection Agency standards.

Our diet contains booster herbs and spices such as garlic, ginger, and shiitake mushrooms, which contain many plant chemicals known to improve immunity and reduce inflammation; ginger also contains a brochodilator.

What About Calcium?

In the United States, we have come to believe that unless a child drinks a lot of milk everyday, she is not getting enough calcium. So you may be wondering: can my child get enough calcium from this diet, which advises against milk and cheese? The answer is yes, if you are confident that your child really is following this diet. This means eating greater than usual amounts of other foods high in calcium, such as green leafy vegetables (spinach, kale, greens of all kinds), salmon and sardines, broccoli, and soybeans and soybean products such as soy milk and tofu. Make sure you buy soy and other nondairy milks fortified with calcium and vitamin D; your child can get about one-quarter of her daily calcium needs from just one cup of fortified soy milk. You also need to make sure she is avoiding foods that deplete calcium from the body, such as sugar, carbonated drinks, caffeine-containing drinks, and excess protein, and she is getting sufficient exercise to build strong healthy bones. There are many studies that show that children in countries that traditionally consume little or no meat or milk grow up to have much less osteoporosis than countries where milk and meat are consumed in large quantities—as long as they eat plenty of vegetables. If your child's diet doesn't meet these criteria, we would be concerned that she is not getting enough calcium; that's why we often recommend a nutritional supplement that contains calcium (see Chapter 7).

THE POWER OF PLANTS

Plants contain a slew of chemicals and compounds that function as *antioxidants*. Antioxidants break the destructive chain of free radical reactions that cause cell damage, inflammation, and asthma (see page 18, Chapter 1). Some of these substances are vitamins—for example vitamins C and E and beta-carotene. Others are known as *phytochemicals*, and more and more of them are being discovered all the time. These include substances in green tea, grape seeds, soybeans, onion and garlic, citrus fruit and citrus fruit peels, broccoli, cabbage, and brussels sprouts.

This may be why Swedish researchers have found that a vegan diet (all plants with no animal products) can reduce symptoms in people with asthma: 90 percent of the subjects studied enjoyed a reduction in the frequency and severity of flare-ups, and 50 percent reduced their medication by at least half, some completely.

ACTION STEP:

SELF-ASSESSMENT QUESTIONNAIRE

This test helps you figure out what your child is really eating and where you need to make changes to bring his diet closer to optimum.

1: Make seven photocopies of this questionnaire and fill it in every day for one week. Refer to the Optimum Diet for details on the specific foods that belong to each food group listed on the questionnaire.

2: To score the test, add up the weekly total in each food group and divide by seven to get the average total per day. Compare the average total number of servings your child eats in each group with those in the Optimum Diet. Then use that as a guide in determining what changes you need to make to improve your child's diet. For example, if your child is eating an average of only one fruit per day, and the optimum amount is 3, the change you need to make is +2.

ACTION STEP:

MAKE GRADUAL CHANGES

Now that you know where your child's diet could stand improvement, the next step is to make the necessary changes. Remember, you are the "gatekeeper"—you control most of what your child eats, at least during early childhood when habits are formed and asthma first occurs. One of the most important things you can do

SELF-ASSESSMENT QUESTIONNAIRE:
WHAT IS YOUR CHILD REALLY EATING?

Date: _____   ••NUMBER OF SERVINGS••

	Brkfst	Lunch	Dinner	Snacks	Total
1. Low Starch Vegetables	___	___	___	___	___
2. Starchy Vegetables	___	___	___	___	___
3. Whole Grains	___	___	___	___	___
4. Fresh Fruit	___	___	___	___	___
5. Beans	___	___	___	___	___
6. Meat, Fish, Poultry	___	___	___	___	___
7. Dairy	___	___	___	___	___
8. Essential Fats	___	___	___	___	___
9. Other Oils	___	___	___	___	___
10. Nuts and Seeds	___	___	___	___	___
11. Booster Herbs and Spices	___	___	___	___	___
12. Water	___	___	___	___	___
13. Processed Foods	___	___	___	___	___

is to set a good example. Which eating habits do you want to pass on to your child? You can change your eating habits so they are healthier for you and you are a better role model for your child. But make changes gradually—any time change is too dramatic, you're likely to meet with resistance and perhaps resentment, making your job much harder.

To help you implement this crucial step, we provide sample menus, tips on preparation, how to deal with obstacles to good eating, and how to accomplish this change in the context of the family and the school environment.

EASING YOUR WAY
TO OPTIMUM EATING

Trying to achieve an optimum diet is a gradual process. Make small changes slowly, rather than sweeping changes that can cause the whole family to rebel. The following tips should smooth out some of the bumps in the road as you move toward a healthier way of eating.

Starting Out

- Begin by placing more emphasis on healthful foods your child already likes. For example, most kids love sweet potatoes, carrots, and berries—foods which are jam-packed with beta-carotene and other beneficial phyto-chemicals. Most kids also like soy cheese, which you can cut into small cubes and add to cooked grains and use in casseroles and cheese melts.

- Don't let your own preferences limit or influence food choices. Many American adults dislike tofu (at least initially), but most children love it, if you present it in a positive or neutral way. Try it crumbled on pizza, in chili, soups, stews, and casseroles. If your child likes meat but not tofu, try some of the new veggie meat substitutes, such as sausage, bacon, deli meats, and hot dogs.

- If your child won't eat whole wheat bread at first, try using whole wheat wraps or whole wheat tortillas.

- Use vegetarian cookbooks to spark up menus with fast, easy dishes. Two of our favorites are *Fresh from a Vegetarian Kitchen* by Meredith McCarty (St. Martin's Press, 1995) and *Moosewood Restaurant Cooks at Home: Fast and Easy Recipes for Any Day* by the Moosewood Collective (Simon and Schuster Books, 1994).

- Involve kids in growing some of their food. Swiss chard, for example, is beautiful to look at and easy to grow; kids will often eat it as a stir-fry. You and your child can make your own sprouts from many grains and seeds such as alfalfa seeds and clover seeds; they are packed with nutrients and are delicious raw or cooked, as a snack or part of a meal.

- If your child has a sweet tooth, you need to work extra hard to find ways to reduce sugary foods. To spark up flavor and make fruit special, try sprinkling lemon juice and cinnamon on apple slices, or nutmeg on peach slices. Buy ginger graham crackers as a sweet treat, or spread all-fruit jams on crackers or matzos which are yeast free. Or try a little bit of plain yogurt mixed with fresh fruit and topped with crunchy Grape Nuts.

- If your child is addicted to juices, try weaning him away gradually by diluting the juice with increasing amounts of water. Iced tea drinks mixed with fruit juices are all the rage, so you may want to try giving your child iced herbal tea containing sweet-tasting herbs such as licorice, which are caffeine free. An excellent choice would be

Breathe Deep Tea by the Yogi Tea Company, containing mild amounts of herbs that open the bronchioles, reduce mucus, reduce lung congestion, and enhance immunity.

Make smoothies. Smoothies are an easy way to introduce several healthful foods into your child's daily diet. Combine fresh fruit chunks (a bit of frozen fruit gives the drink more texture and variety and makes it seem more like store-bought smoothies), nondairy milk, and a teaspoon of flaxseed oil in a blender. This makes a terrific breakfast and, if you make extra to leave in the refrigerator, your child can reach for this instead of a less healthful snack when he gets home from school.

Preparation and Cooking

- Make preparation a pleasure. Vegetable-oriented cooking and preparation can be time consuming. Lighten your burden and get your kids "invested" in their food by having them help with the preparation. Even a five-year-old child can set the table or scrub some vegetables—and help you come up with appealing ways to prepare and present new foods.

- Make life easy—take advantage of labor-saving advances such as precut and prewashed salads and raw vegetables in resealable bags.

- Be sneaky. One of the hardest things to get into kids is leafy greens and green vegetables, so sneak these and other healthy foods into favorite dishes. For example, add escarole or other deep greens to a white bean soup. Serve pureed soups; for example, broccoli, potatoes, and onions make a marvelous combination. The parents of one of our patients came up with a new name for pureed soups—"pretty soup"—which the father made as a special treat.

- It is best to steam, bake, or broil foods, without added fat. Steaming vegetables until tender yet still bright in color preserves their nutrients better than boiling or overcooking. Sautéing in a small amount of oil is also acceptable. Try dressing up steamed vegetables with a dollop of mild salsa or melted cheddar soy cheese.

- Emphasize colorful foods and foods your child can pick up with his fingers; broccoli spears, carrot sticks, red bell peppers, melon balls, quartered sandwiches, and sliced wraps are especially appealing to young children.

- Simple dishes are better than complicated recipes with lots of ingredients. Kids like to be able to see clearly what it is they are eating.

- Wraps, burritos, and corn tortillas are also kid-friendly ways to introduce more vegetables and beans into your child's diet.

- To include garlic in your child's diet, sneak it into your favorite homemade soup by using garlic broth as a base. To make the broth, smash and peel three whole heads of garlic and sauté over low heat in one tablespoon olive oil for twenty minutes until soft; do not let it get brown. Add two quarts of water and bring to a boil; let simmer for forty minutes. Cooking garlic this way makes it mild and sweet. To make soup, add your own favorite tasty vegetables and spices, such as peas and carrots, onions, spinach, potatoes, tomatoes, or a handful of immune-boosting fresh or dried shiitake or maitake mushrooms.

- To include ginger in your child's diet, grate fresh ginger root and add to sautéed vegetables. Add a few drops to fresh fruit juices. Another way your child might like the taste is in ginger tea. Our favorite method of making ginger tea is to take a piece of fresh ginger root the size of a checker. Peel the tough outer skin and cut into smaller pieces. Put 6 ounces of water in a blender and start it whirring; then drop in the ginger until blended. Pour into a saucepan and bring to a boil; add 1 teaspoon honey to sweeten, if desired; you may also add lemon juice if you wish. One cup per day is ideal as prevention, and your child may drink more during a flare-up.

- Try this nutritious sauce as a vegetable dip, salad dressing, or flavoring for a steaming bowl of whole grains. Blend at medium speed: 1/2 pound of soft or silken tofu, 1 tablespoon sesame tahini, 1 tablespoon miso (soybean paste), 1/2 cup plain yogurt (optional), 1 tablespoon lemon juice, soy sauce to taste. You can vary this recipe with herbs and spices. This keeps refrigerated for one week.

- Use glass or stainless steel cookware and avoid coated cookware which can contaminate foods with unwanted chemicals.

- Avoid using a microwave because there is evidence that microwaves break delicate chemical bonds in foods, and microwave ovens tend to leak electromagnetic radiation, which may be harmful.

Eating in the Real World

- If your child eats lunch at school, encourage him to make choices based on the optimum diet. Get a doctor's note explaining your child's requirements—the school food service is legally required to provide the special diet your child needs. Better yet, prepare your child's lunch (have him make it at home) using the substitutes mentioned earlier in this chapter—whole wheat bread instead of white, soy cheese instead of dairy cheese.

- Kids are bound to hang out with their buddies at candy stores, the mall, and convenience stores that sell fast foods. Just do the best you can. Make sure your child is well supplied with healthy snacks to carry along with him.

- If you have a young child attending day care or preschool, be ready for parties and celebrations by bringing allowed snack foods for your child and remind the staff to give them to your child discreetly.

- Relatives' and friends' homes can be difficult. Talk to them, encourage them to be supportive of your efforts, give them a list of foods that are healthy for your child, or show them this book.

- Negotiate with your child so he doesn't feel deprived. One mother says, "We go easy on the wheat—our son isn't allergic per se, but most people's diets include wheat at every meal. That's too much of one thing. It's the same thing with dairy. What we do is, for example, Fridays are pizza days at school. Our son can have the wheat crust, and the cheese. But he can't have an ice cream cone afterwards. If we were going to go out that night for ice cream, he knows he has to get the peanut butter and jelly sandwich for lunch instead."

- Halloween candy poses unique challenges, especially if your child is allergic. Trick or treat candies often do not have ingredient labels and are laden with sugar. To minimize problems, deliver acceptable treats to your neighbors' homes before the festivities begin; for example, raisins, pretzels, mini rice crackers, and nonedible treats such as stickers. Explain to your child beforehand that he or she may need to trade certain candies with friends or with you. Finally, you can accompany your child as he makes his rounds to be sure that he doesn't inadvertently eat harmful candies.

Shopping

- Favor fresh fruits and vegetables, locally grown, in season. If fresh is not available, choose frozen vegetables or fruit, without preservatives or additives. Avoid canned produce.

- Look for convenient grain mixes with packets of herbs that cook in about a half hour.

- To avoid food additives, read labels and don't eat anything with an ingredient whose name you don't recognize or can't pronounce.

- To cut down on sugar, emphasize fresh fruit instead of baked goods and candy. Whole baby carrots may help appease your child's sweet tooth and are rich in fiber and essential nutrients.

- Watch out for fruit juice, which seems healthful but is actually a poor choice because it is not a whole food. They are a concentrated source of sugar, are low in fiber, and low in nutrients unless consumed immediately after juicing. Commercial juices, though better for your child than additive-laden sodas, are still to be avoided.

- If your child doesn't like the grainy texture of whole-wheat pasta, try pastas made with half whole wheat and half white flour, such as those made by Eden (800-

248-0301). Good whole-grain cereals are made by Barbara's Bakery (800-747-0390).

SHOULD YOU EAT ORGANIC?

We recommend that our patients buy organic produce if possible. Although it is still more expensive than conventionally grown produce, it is becoming more available. According to *Fresh Trends* magazine, approximately half of all supermarkets offer organic produce. The reasons to go organic are compelling. It's been estimated that eight-hundred million pounds of pesticides are used annually on farms. Some of this inevitably winds up in your child's body through the food he eats, adding to the toxic burden. In addition, according to a recent report in *The Journal of Applied Nutrition*, organic fruits and vegetables are up to twice as rich in some nutrients than conventionally grown produce. They also often have a better taste and texture than conventional, and thus children are more likely to eat them. That's why we recommend buying produce that has been grown organically. And make sure meat and dairy products come from animals that have been raised organically, if you eat them.

If cost is an issue, buy foods in bulk and split the cost with other parents. Look for a food buying co-op or a farmer's market. If organic food is still too costly or unavailable for you, consider switching to organic for the worst offenders. According to the organization Mothers and Others for a Livable Planet, the ten most contaminated foods—and hence, the most important foods to buy in organic form—are baby food, strawberries, rice, milk, corn, bananas, green beans, peaches, apples, and oats and other grains. And minimizing or eliminating meat and meat products will also help, because animals are high on the food chain, which means pesticides and other toxins accumulate in their cells and thus offer a concentrated source of these harmful chemicals.

If you buy conventionally grown and raised food, the Environmental Protection Agency has issued a brochure that provides suggestions for reducing pesticide residues in food. These include: washing and scrubbing fruits and vegetables under running water, peeling and trimming fruits and vegetables, and trimming the fat from meat and poultry.

Other Suggestions

- If your child is picky and eats just a few things, rewarding him with dessert if he eats his vegetables will only reinforce finicky behavior. Rather, praising him with words, especially when other people are around, works best.

- Encourage your child to become involved in improving his diet, to be aware of foods that are helpful and those that are harmful and to take responsibility for the food he eats.

- You can't control what his friends' parents keep in their homes, but you can choose what to keep in yours, so don't keep junk food in your home. Keep plenty of healthy foods available for snacking such as baby carrots, fruits such as grapes and berries, and rice cakes.

- If your child is overweight, serve smaller portions and emphasize foods recommended in the Optimum Diet.

- Encourage your child to exercise because it improves digestion and absorption of nutrients. Exercise is also important for children who are overweight because it burns calories and decreases appetite. (See Chapter 4 for information on exercise and asthma.)

- Limit TV watching, which is a sedentary activity peppered with commercials that coax your child to eat processed foods. It is estimated that the average child watches twenty-five hours of TV a week; 15 percent of that is commercials; and of that, 70 percent is commercials for food—that works out to two and one-half hours of junk food commercials a week .

SUGAR SURPRISE

Excess sugar can harm your child's immune system. You'd be surprised at the amount of sugar in common foods that many children eat and drink regularly:

12 ounces of colas and sodas . . . . . 7–9 teaspoons

1 ounce of fudge. . . . . 4–5 teaspoons

1/2 cup ice cream . . . . 5 teaspoons

Even foods we consider to be healthy or not that sweet contain a surprising amount of sugar:

1/2 cup canned fruit cocktail . . . . 5 teaspoons

12 ounces apple cider . . . . 6 teaspoons

2 tablespoons jam . . . . 4–6 teaspoons

1 cup cocoa . . . . 4 teaspoons

ACTION STEP:

TREAT FOOD ALLERGIES AND SENSITIVITIES

If professional allergy testing or the daily diary you are keeping for your child suggests he might be sensitive to food, making the changes needed to feed your child the Optimum Diet will not be sufficient. The Optimum Diet will still be the framework, but you will need to modify it by eliminating the foods that act as a trigger for your child.

There are several ways your child may be adversely reacting to food. He may have a classic allergic reaction. This type of reaction involves the immune system chemical immunoglobulin E and is well understood and widely recognized. Or your child may be sensitive or intolerant to certain foods. These abnormal reactions do not involve the same immune system mechanisms as in a classic allergy. They may involve a substance called immunoglobulin G or another mechanism entirely. Conventional allergists tend to ignore or overlook many of these types of nonclassic allergic reactions. We believe this is a big mistake: only one-third of food allergies involve immunoglobulin E; the remaining involve IgG or other mechanisms.

In our centers, we have found that it is extremely common for children with asthma to experience adverse food reactions. In fact, *most* of the children we treat have food allergies or sensitivities. Once we treat children for food reactions, their asthma improves and they become less sensitive to other allergens that are less controllable, such as pollen.

Food allergies or sensitivities can trigger asthma in a number of ways. A food particle may leak from the digestive system into the bloodstream without being fully digested, and the immune system sees this harmless food particle as a potential invader. White blood cells, blood vessels, and even distant organs such as the adrenal glands respond by releasing a torrent of biochemicals including histamines, which produce allergic symptoms. Allergic reaction or asthma symptoms can be within minutes or hours after your child eats the offending food, as the inflammatory chemicals build up in the body and affect the hypersensitive lungs.

Allergies to foods can trigger a variety of symptoms including gastrointestinal symptoms, hives or other skin reactions such as eczema, difficulty swallowing, headache, anxiety, fatigue, mood swings, joint pain, irritable bowel syndrome, and migraine. Many of our patients with chronic asthma find that their problems lessen or even disappear if they simply avoid dairy products.

There is a small group of foods that cause the most problems. The foods most commonly linked to asthma episodes are milk, eggs, and soy and wheat products. Sulfites, common food additives, have also been linked with asthma flare-ups. We find that eliminating these foods from a child's diet most often reduces symptoms dramatically. Since food allergies can be delayed, even if your daily diary doesn't definitively indicate that these foods may be a problem, we recommend that you try the following elimination diet.

At-Home Elimination Diet

This is the simplest way to determine whether your child has food sensitivities.

- Do not feed your child the foods listed as the top six foods to eliminate for eight to nine days. If you suspect any foods listed under other common food allergens, also eliminate them from the diet for that time.

- Continue to keep a daily diary to see if symptoms improve.

- If symptoms do improve after seven to fourteen days, determine the specific foods to which she is most sensitive by reintroducing one food at a time, every other day, to see if symptoms return. If they do, that food is a trigger; continue to avoid that food as much as possible. (You may want to try reintroducing it again after three months to see if she is still sensitive.) If symptoms do not return after reintroducing a specific food, you may continue to include that food in her regular diet.

- If you do not see any improvement, and you still suspect food allergies may be a trigger for your child, consult a professional with expertise in food allergies.

Top Six Foods to Eliminate:

- *Milk and Dairy Products:* Cow's milk and milk products such as cream, ice cream, ice milk, yogurt, cheese, lactose, casein or caseinate, whey, lactoglobulin, albumin, milk solids. Substitute plant-derived milks such as soy, rice, almond, and oatmeal, available at health food stores and an increasing number of grocery stores.

- *Eggs:* Eggs and products containing eggs. Use egg substitutes for home cooking, but read labels carefully, as some egg substitutes contain egg white.

- *Soy:* Soy products such as tofu, soy milk, cheese, yogurt, burgers, and hot dogs.

- *Wheat:* Wheat products such as bread, muffins, crackers, cereals, pastries, pasta, cookies, cakes, pizza, pretzels, couscous. Wheat may appear on labels as wheat flour, graham flour, malt, bran, wheat germ, gluten, farina, or wheat starch thickeners.

- *Gluten-containing foods:* These include wheat, oats, and rye.

- *Sulfites:* Foods likely to contain sulfites, used as a preservative, include: shrimp; frozen, canned, or dried fruits and vegetables; wine and wine vinegar; beer; fruit drinks; potato chips; baked goods; processed foods. Sulfites are also found in many medications including bronchodilating medications used in nebulizers. Many children are also affected by additives such as thickeners, flavor enhancers, food coloring, pesticides residues, and preservatives.

Other Common Food Allergens:

- Peanuts and foods containing peanuts.
- Fish and shellfish, including shrimp and lobster.

- Chocolate and chocolate-containing products.
- Mold-containing foods: baked goods with yeast as the leavening agent; cheese; dried fruits; mushrooms; soy sauce; vinegar and foods that contain vinegar such as pickles, ketchup, salad dressings, mayonnaise, relish, and sauerkraut; smoked meats including sausage, hot dogs, and corned beef; buttermilk; sour cream; beer, wine, or cider.

Adopting a Hypoallergenic Diet

Eating an optimum diet is challenging enough; if your child has food allergies, it adds another layer of complexity. We have found the following suggestions to be most helpful to our patients in dealing with the three primary challenges to following a hypoallergenic diet.

- *Use Substitutes.* Parents with allergic children find it especially challenging to avoid the more common foods such as milk and wheat because they are in so many foods. But as the awareness of food sensitivities grows, so does the availability of substitutes. For example, health-food stores and supermarkets with large health-food sections sell many nonwheat flours, grains, and baked goods, as well as pastas. There are now many dairy-free ice creams, yogurts, milks, and cheeses. Carob is a widely available chocolate substitute. We find that although it may take some time for children to get used to these foods, the taste and texture of these foods are improving all the time. For example, it's now possible to prepare melted cheddar soy cheese sandwiches on amaranth bread, followed by a frozen carob rice milk dessert.

- *Be creative and adventurous.* There are many allergy cookbooks and cookbooks on vegetarian cooking that offer new, delicious ways to use unfamiliar ingredients. Recipes can be quite simple—just a matter of combining foods in a refreshing way. For example, babies and toddlers love the taste and texture of the grain quinoa, which is delicious mixed with mashed sweet potatoes. Buckwheat and string beans makes a protein-packed, fiber-filled dish with a delicious nutty flavor. The mother of one of our patients was dismayed to discover that her daughter was allergic to peanuts, and peanut butter and jelly sandwiches were commonly served at her school for lunch. She cleverly used hummus (chickpea puree) to make sandwiches and left them with the teacher to give to her child later in the day. The hummus resembled peanut butter closely enough so her child did not feel like an outcast during lunch.

- *Read labels carefully.* Another challenge is in avoiding hidden ingredients. Be sure to scrutinize labels of packaged foods carefully, because you'll be surprised at how many foods contain wheat, soy, milk, and eggs. You may discover a few surprises, too: Some egg substitutes contain egg white, and some nondairy creamers contain milk. And you must continue to check labels, even if you buy the same product, because manufacturers change their contents regularly. You can avoid a lot of the label hassle by making your own "convenience foods": Start with fresh, pure ingredients and make casseroles, soups, stews, and other freezables in large batches to defrost and use as needed.

<u>PRECAUTION:</u> Do not use this diet without medical supervision if your child suffers from severe allergies and may go into anaphylactic shock when exposed to a particu-

lar allergen. If your child has severe asthma, we also recommend that you consult a professional for guidance. In our practice, we frequently give the child nutritional supplements to strengthen his constitution before undergoing the elimination diet, as the withdrawal symptoms and elimination of so many toxins can be too taxing for an unfortified body.

Preventing Allergic Asthma

Whether a child develops allergies and asthma depends on genetic predisposition and upon whatever they are exposed to during infancy, early childhood, and even in the womb. You can't change genetic makeup and predisposition to asthma, but you can reduce the risk of your child becoming sensitized to allergens. Exposure early in life seems to be the key—when they are most vulnerable. So if you already have one child with asthma and have younger children or are thinking of having more, following these guidelines will reduce the risk of another child becoming sensitized to common substances and developing this condition.

1: When pregnant, eat a well-balanced, nutritious diet and avoid bingeing on any one food.

2: Breast-feed for at least the first year because this reduces the risk of allergies as well as protects from respiratory infections and ear infections. In highly allergic families, we usually recommend that the nursing mothers avoid dairy products, soy, corn, wheat, and eggs because these proteins can be passed to the baby through the mother's milk.

3: Do not give your baby solid food for the first six months; the fewer the number of foods introduced at this time, the better. We recommend you follow this schedule for introducing foods; it begins with the least allergenic foods:

- 7 months: introduce small amounts of vegetables and rice cereals.
- 8 months: gradually begin increasing the amount of rice.
- 9 months: if you wish, begin introducing small amounts of meat; avoid fish at this time.
- 10 months: introduce noncitrus fruits.
- 12 months: add other grains such as millet, rye, oats, and wheat; beans and lentils; corn; citrus fruits.
- Avoid highly allergenic foods such as eggs, peanuts, chocolate, fish, strawberries, and nuts for the first year.
- As you introduce new foods, do so slowly, one at a time, no more than one per week, and watch closely for signs of allergy such as rash, stomach upset, cough, breathing problems.
- Follow the suggestions we provide in Chapter 4 for avoiding triggers for all children, not just the child who already has asthma. Most importantly, do not expose your child to smoke—yours or anyone else's.

ACTION STEP:

WORKING WITH A HEALTH PROFESSIONAL

Working with a professional to get a balanced, nutritious diet is especially helpful if your child has multiple food allergies or delayed reactions. In these cases, it may simply be too difficult for you to identify the food or foods that are causing the reactions. So, if your child still has symptoms after eliminating the obvious offenders, or if he is a picky eater who refuses to eat healing foods, don't give up. Consider seeking professional guidance.

At our health centers, we have a certified nutritionist on staff. We would recommend that you consult with someone who has similar credentials or a nutritionally oriented physician.

When you work with a knowledgeable professional, you will get more ideas on how to change eating habits for the better, extensive menu ideas, recipes, and shopping tips. You and your child will also benefit from more sophisticated tools for determining food allergies, such as the double-blind test in which neither you nor the doctor nor your child knows what food is being tested. You will get more detailed knowledge about foods to avoid if your child is allergic to corn, for example, or needs to avoid yeast because of a yeast allergy or because of an overgrowth of yeast in the body.

A professional may prescribe a diet consisting of a limited group of specific foods that rarely cause allergic reactions. These usually consist of lamb, turkey, rice, carrots, pears, and sweet potatoes for one week. Parents then gradually introduce new foods ("challenge"), one at a time every three days, and monitor for allergic reactions using a food diary. The elimination/challenge diet helps detoxify and identify an individual child's particular triggers, so parents can fine-tune and individualize the daily diet. In our clinic, we regularly recommend that our patients use a special hypoallergenic powder to make a tasty shake to supplement this limited diet, which makes it easy to avoid wheat, corn, and milk and encourages the detoxification process.

Eating an optimum diet, tailored to any food allergies your child may have, is the foundation of a nutritionally-oriented asthma prevention program. Once you have followed this type of diet as part of the Natural Asthma Control Program explained in Chapter 4, you are ready to progress to a more intensive level of nutritional therapy involving supplements geared specifically towards controlling asthma.

SEVEN

NUTRITIONAL SUPPLEMENTS

Eating according to the guidelines in the previous chapter will go a long way towards keeping asthma symptoms at bay. But unfortunately it is unlikely that even an optimum diet will supply your child with enough vitamins, minerals, and other key nutrients needed to foster optimum health, let alone take care of hypersensitive airways and inflammation. That's why at our health centers we seldom stop with dietary recommendations. We have seen first-hand—in our patients, in ourselves, and in our families—the additional benefits of taking nutritional supplements. No Natural Asthma Control Program is complete without at least a moderate amount of supplementation, in addition to eating the Optimum Diet outlined in the previous chapter.

In this chapter we explain why supplementation is becoming increasingly accepted and recommended for children with asthma. Then you'll learn which specific nutrients, and what amounts, have been found to be the most beneficial for asthma and immune function. This is followed by a section on how to use supplements for optimum health, asthma prevention, and symptom relief. In addition, this chapter provides a primer on how to buy, store, and take supplements as well as what precautions to take and what to expect from a nutrition specialist.

REMINDER: When you take any of the steps in this chapter, remember to continue your child's regular medical treatment. Do not reduce asthma medications on your own—do this only under the advice and supervision of your child's physician. If your child shows any of the danger signs of an asthma flare-up (see page 59, Chapter 4), seek medical attention immediately.

WHY USE SUPPLEMENTS?

While a nutritious diet is still the mainstay of good health, this is not always possible to achieve. As we have seen in the previous chapter, it takes planning and effort to eat an optimum diet. Supplements offer a type of insurance for those days when you simply cannot get at least five servings of fresh fruits and vegetables into your child, and you settle for toaster pop-ups for breakfast, pizza for lunch, or burgers for dinner.

Many studies and surveys have shown that it's a rare child indeed who obtains from food alone what we consider to be the bare minimum of nutrients—the Food and Drug Administration's Recommended Daily Allowances (RDAs). The RDAs were established by the National Academy of Sciences to provide a safety margin for essential nutrients that would prevent deficiency diseases such as scurvy, pellagra, and beriberi. (Recently, the RDAs were replaced by the RDIs, Reference Daily Intakes, which represent the *average* need; they are essentially the same as the RDAs.) That's why it's wise to take a daily vitamin-mineral formula that supplies *at least* the RDA for all the known vitamins and minerals.

But recent studies show that the RDAs are not enough for optimum health. Although the RDAs were a significant step in improving nutrition in this country, many respected authorities no longer believe the RDAs are really adequate for every person. The RDAs often fall far short of creating and maintaining optimum health, nor are they adequate if a person has health problems such as asthma and is trying to get better.

In addition, the RDAs are a "one-size-fits-all" approach. But all children are not alike. They are born with their own unique biological blueprints which include individual nutrient requirements and predisposition to diseases such as asthma. In addition, children today are under an unprecedented amount of physical stress from a polluted environment and psychological stress from their complicated, hectic lives. Such stresses are known to deplete the body of nutrients, and supplemental nutrients help protect the lungs, immune system, and other systems against damage from such stresses. Furthermore, drugs such as steroids, nonsteroidals, and antibiotics affect nutrient absorption and requirements. For example, steroids deplete the body of calcium, antioxidants, chromium, and magnesium. Nutritional supplements in optimum amounts higher than the RDA can make up the difference.

There are many exciting new studies that show that higher amounts of certain nutrients, such as beta-carotene, vitamin E, and vitamin C, have many beneficial effects. These amounts are impossible to get from food or from low-dose supplements containing just the RDAs. We'll go into the benefits of specific nutrients later in this chapter, but in summation, studies suggest that higher-than-RDA amounts of certain nutrients can:

- Detoxify
- Protect the respiratory system
- Reduce unnecessary inflammation
- Improve resistance to infection
- Stabilize the immune system
- Relieve specific symptoms

ACTION STEP:

SUPPLEMENTS FOR ASTHMA PREVENTION

Although certain nutrients appear to be the most beneficial for asthma, as a general rule it's best not to take a supplement containing just one nutrient or a few nutrients. Nutrients typically work synergistically and frequently depend on one another to work efficiently. For example, the B vitamins usually work best together. In addition, taking large doses of one nutrient can create an imbalance in your body. For example, you may think it wise to give your child vitamin B-6 because it has been shown to relax the airways. However, if you take only vitamin B-6 it will compete with other B vitamins to be absorbed in the intestine, and an excess of B-6 could create a deficiency in the others.

That is why the "Optimum Daily Amounts" chart below gives the recommended dosages for the full spectrum of the best-known nutrients in amounts that are safe for children. The lowest number is the amount we generally recommend to our patients for general optimum health and for asthma prevention. The simplest way to begin this step of the program is to give your child a complete multi-vitamin-mineral supplement formula that comes closest to this lower amount. There are several children's formulas (and for teenagers, adult formulas) that approximate these amounts. However, you may need to add single supplements of flavonoids and vitamins C and E to reach optimum amounts. You will also need to buy separate supplements of garlic and omega-3 fatty acids.

Be sure to buy a supplement that requires that your child take several tablets two or three times a day—supplements work best when doses are divided throughout the day. To minimize any adverse reactions such as an upset stomach, for the first two weeks give your child half the recommended dosage specified on the label. If possible, divide this over the course of the day. For example, if the dosage is two tablets two times a day, give her one tablet two times a day. Then increase it to the full recommended dosage. Children tend to dislike taking pills, so we recommend opening up capsules and adding them to food, or buying chewable supplements.

Because they need to become part of the cells of your child's body, it takes time for supplements to have a noticeable effect. You may see some improvement in as little as two weeks; continue to expect improvement in the months to come. If you do not see improvement after three months, increase the dosage to the higher number on the chart, which is the therapeutic level, after consulting with a nutritionally-oriented physician or other qualified nutrition expert. As your child's health improves, you may be able to lower the dosages over time to the maintenance level. If you still do not see any improvement, consult with your nutrition professional.

Remember, nutritional supplements are just that—*supplements* to a healthful, balanced diet and active lifestyle, not *substitutes*. Taking supplements is not a license to let your child slip off the Optimum Diet.

A Parent's Guide to Using Supplements

When buying, using, and storing supplements, keep in mind:

- Buy supplements that contain little or no inert ingredients such as fillers and artificial flavors and colors because these can add to the toxic burden.

- Buy hypoallergenic supplements that contain no yeast, corn, wheat, soy, milk, or egg. Your child could have hidden allergies to these substances.

- Store supplements in a cool, dark, dry place—not the refrigerator, which is damp. (The exception is essential fatty oils such as flaxseed oil, which require refrigeration.) Supplements have a limited shelf life, so toss them after the expiration date.

- Try to divide the dosage throughout the day to increase effectiveness. For example, if your child is taking 450 mg of vitamin C, give her 150 mg three times a day.

- Take most supplements with meals; this also increases absorption and prevents indigestion or "tasting" the vitamins later.

OPTIMUM DAILY AMOUNTS

We generally recommend the following dosages:

- children aged 6–12 and who are 45" to 57" tall—full dosages
- children aged 12 and up and 57" tall or more —double the dosages
- children aged 2–6 and from 34" to 45" in height —roughly half the dosages
- children ages 1–2—consult with a nutritional professional

Nutrient	General Maintenance	Therapeutic*
Vitamin A	5,000 IU	5,000 IU
Beta-carotene	5,000 IU	5,000 IU–10,000 IU
Vitamin B-1	10 mg	20 mg
B-2	5 mg	10 mg
B-3	20 mg	40 mg
B-6	10 mg	20 mg
B-12	100 mcg	100 mcg
Folic acid	300 mcg	600 mcg
Pantothenic acid	100 mg	300–500 mg
Biotin	150 mcg	150 mcg
Vitamin C	100	500 mg+
Vitamin D	100 IU	200 IU
Vitamin E	100 IU	200 IU
Calcium	250 mg	250 mg
Magnesium	250 mg	250–400 mg
Selenium	50 mcg	100 mcg
Zinc	10 mg	10–20 mg
Copper	1 mg	1–2 mg
Omega-3	250mg	500–1,000 mg
Flavonoids	100mg	200–300 mg
Garlic	1-3 (350 mg) capsules	1–3 (350 mg) capsules
N-acetylcysteine (NAC)	500 mg	500 mg
**Iron	1 mg per year of age	1 mg per year of age

* Consult with a nutritionally oriented physician before taking these amounts. Some supplements may interact with medication or cause adverse reactions. The recommended dosages have been found to be safe in the vast majority of children; however, be alert for any possible side effects or unusual sensitivities.

** For iron, take a separate supplement; do not rely on a multiformula.

THE BENEFITS OF NUTRIENTS

Now that you know *what* to give your child, you will want to have a more detailed explanation of *why* we believe these nutrients in these amounts are beneficial. What follows is a summary of the most beneficial nutrients for asthma.

As you'll see, the various nutrients have many functions, but one of the most important functions shared by a variety of nutrients is that of *antioxidant*. As you read in the previous chapter, eating plant foods is an excellent way of getting antioxidants— including those we have not yet discovered and thus cannot be found in a pill. However, supplements are the only way to get generous amounts of the known antioxidants.

Antioxidants are the most important type of supplement for children with asthma because they support health in many ways. Antioxidants help neutralize toxins and free radicals, protecting cells from damage caused by exposure to pollution, poor diet, medication, and stress and from natural metabolic processes such as inflammation. Remember, inflammation is at the root of asthma, and if cells should become damaged, antioxidants also help damaged cells repair themselves and regenerate. Antioxidants help regulate the immune system so it is neither overreactive (which would provoke allergies and inflammation) nor underreactive (which would increase susceptibility to infection).

Antioxidants include vitamin C, vitamin E, beta-carotene, selenium, zinc, and glutathione. Antioxidant enzymes include superoxide dismutase and glutathione peroxidase; to function, these require certain vitamin, mineral, and amino acid cofactors.

Most of the positive studies using supplements involve the antioxidant nutrients vitamins E, C, and A and beta-carotene, and the minerals zinc and selenium. These studies suggest that doses *in excess* of the RDA for these antioxidant nutrients are particularly useful in enhancing immunity and reducing the risk of infection, allergy, and asthma. When you give your child antioxidants, studies suggest, you are also reducing her risk of many other conditions including cancer and heart disease.

Antioxidants work together in the body to replenish each other and increase each other's effectiveness. The best strategy for boosting immune function and preventing asthma is to take all the known antioxidants along with the full spectrum of other vitamins and minerals.

Vitamin A and Beta-carotene

Vitamin A and its precursor, beta-carotene, are antioxidants. They are needed by your child's immune system because they help stimulate production of antibodies, T-cells, and natural killer cells that fight infection and cancer. Vitamin A also maintains epithelial cells and mucus membranes in the respiratory system—physical barriers that serve as your child's first line of defense against invasion by harmful substances that might trigger asthma or lead to infection. Beta-carotene helps the body detoxify smoke and other air pollutants and modulates the release of prostaglandins and leukotrienes, anti-inflammatory chemicals. Unlike many other nutrients, it is possible to get high amounts of beta-carotene from diet alone, and in food they are accompanied by the other beneficial carotenes. You may, therefore, prefer to rely on food—orange and yellow fruits and vegetables such as winter squash, carrots, and cantaloupe—or feed these foods to your child but give her beta-carotene supplements in addition.

B Vitamins

B-complex vitamins are used by your body to produce immune system components: T-cells, B-cells, antibodies, and other immune-system proteins. All the B vitamins, B-1 (thiamin), B-2 (riboflavin), B-3 (niacin), B-6 (pyridoxine), B-12 (cobalamin), folic acid, pantothenic acid, biotin, choline, inositol, and PABA (para-aminobenzoic acid) work together in the body and are needed for many functions. Vitamin B-6 is especially beneficial for children with asthma because in several studies, supplements of this vitamin have been found to relax the bronchi. In a study involving seventy-six children two to sixteen years old, those taking 200 mg daily experienced less frequent asthma flare-ups, less wheezing, less chest tightness, and easier breathing; they also needed less medication. We don't recommend such high doses for children, unless working under professional supervision.

Vitamin C

Vitamin C is a known antioxidant that protects the watery parts of cells from free radical damage. Furthermore, it regenerates the antioxidant vitamin E after it has neutralized free radicals; it also increases the levels of glutathione in the tissues. This multipurpose vitamin helps the body convert toxins into harmless substances. Studies show that vitamin C is needed to maintain collagen, the protein that gives skin, tendon, bone, cartilage, and connective tissue their structure—remember, a strong respiratory tract is your child's first defense against asthma triggers including viral and bacterial infection. Vitamin C is also an anti-inflammatory and antihistamine, important attributes in treating asthma. In fact, when 300 mg of vitamin C were given to people during an asthma episode, some got instant relief and others got relief within an hour. Another study by the same researchers showed that 150 mg of vitamin C per day were able to prevent asthma flare-ups in some people.

Vitamin C, also called ascorbic acid, is well known as an immunity enhancer. In this capacity it stimulates the production of lymphocytes; is required by the thymus gland, which produces T-cells; increases the effects of phagocytes, which "eat" bacteria, viral cells, and cancer cells; increases levels of interferon; and quiets the effects of a stress hormone, cortisol, which dampens immunity and increases susceptibility to infections which may trigger asthma.

There are many laboratory (test-tube) studies in which vitamin C has inactivated a variety of viruses and bacteria, and levels of vitamin C in white cells drop when we have colds or other infections. There are over twenty studies that show that vitamin C supplements may not be able to prevent a cold or flu, but that when taken in large amounts, they can ease symptoms and shorten a cold's duration. In addition, vitamin C reduces spasms in the airways and is especially useful in preventing asthma symptoms before exercise.

Vitamin E

Vitamin E is a potent antioxidant and protects the fatty parts of cell membranes in particular. It works together with selenium. This vitamin has been shown to enhance almost every aspect of the immune system—resistance to infection, antibody response, and the activity of lymphocytes and phagocytes, all of which are related to asthma prevention. Other studies suggest that vitamin E is needed to maintain healthy macrophages, T-cells, and B-cells. Vitamin E protects against environmental toxins, thus reducing your child's toxic load. It is an anti-inflammatory since it inhibits the production of inflammatory prostaglandins.

Magnesium

This mineral has many functions including immune system function. It helps to stabilize the mast cells so they do not release histamine. A deficiency in magnesium also encourages the production of free radicals and their damaging effects on fats in particular. Both of these functions are involved in inflammation, the underlying cause of asthma. But the most compelling reason for magnesium supplementation as asthma treatment is due to the role it plays in muscle function. Science has known for over fifty years that magnesium is a potent natural brochodilator. It relaxes the smooth muscle and quickly opens up the airways. It is now administered intravenously in hospitals along with medications to treat acute asthma episodes, and we do this at our health centers too. We also recommend daily oral magnesium supplements, preferably in liquid form, as part of a prevention plan and to reduce incidence of nighttime spasms. We sometimes recommend a supplement that combines magnesium with calcium. There are two reasons for this. One, because these two minerals must be taken in correct proportion to each other and two, if children who are not drinking milk are also not eating enough calcium-rich vegetables, they run the risk of being deficient in this mineral.

Selenium

This mineral is itself an antioxidant—and it activates glutathione peroxidase, an antioxidant enzyme produced by the body. Studies show that selenium supplementation activates phagocytes and is anti-inflammatory, which helps prevent asthma. This mineral is known as an anticancer mineral because so many studies equate high intakes or blood levels with a lower rate of many types of cancer.

Zinc

Zinc acts as a cofactor for over three hundred enzyme systems and is required for many processes in the body, including cell growth, normal development, and wound healing. It is required, along with copper, to form the antioxidant enzyme superoxide dismutase. In its role as an immune supporter, it increases circulating lymphocytes and increases antibody production. This mineral is depleted during upper respiratory infections when they are accompanied by fever. Many studies show that zinc boosts immunity, and recently health professionals have been recommending zinc supplements to reduce symptoms during a cold. No one knows for certain why zinc reduces symptoms. But there are several theories: Zinc seems to inhibit the virus from reproducing; it may prevent the virus from entering the cell; it appears to step up production of interferon; and it also may reduce inflammation. So, zinc may prevent and reduce asthma by reducing inflammation and helping to prevent and treat upper respiratory infections.

Other Nutrients

Supplements of other substances that are not quite vitamins or minerals may also help build immunity, reduce inflammation, help detoxify, and repel colds and flu. Among the most studied are:

Flavonoids:

A group of plant chemicals that are antioxidants; they are also anti-inflammatory, antiallergic, and antiviral. Flavonoids prevent the release of histamine and reduce reactivity in allergic children, as well as decrease muscle spasms in the lungs. The best-known flavonoids include quercetin, which helps to stabilize mast cells and prevent the release of histamine and is an antioxidant, and proanthocyanidins (also sometimes called pycnogenols), which are potent antioxidants that have antiallergy and anti-inflammatory effects. We recommend a supplement of mixed flavonoids for most children.

Omega-3:

An essential fatty acid that is anti-inflammatory and enhances immunity. It seems to be especially important in reducing the underlying chronic inflammation that is the cause of chronic asthma and the resulting tissue damage. (See page 108 in Chapter 6 for more basic information about fatty acids.) We usually recommend fish oil in capsule form as the most potent supplement source; look for capsules that have been prepared using an improved process that prevents children from burping up the fishy taste. One type of omega-3 called DHA can be chewed as well as swallowed. We then may switch them to flaxseed oil, which has no aftertaste. Some children respond to borage oil or evening primrose oil, sources of gammalinoleic acid (GLA), another essential fatty acid that indirectly dampens inflammation. Although powerful anti-inflammatories, omega-3 fatty acids may take several months to undo tissue damage and have a significant noticeable effect. **(Note: do not give fish oil to a child who is sensitive to aspirin.)**

Garlic:

A food that contains an impressive concentration of antioxidants, vitamins, and minerals. It has a long history as medicine—this potent anti-infective was used as long ago as 3000 B.C., in ancient Greece. It is antibacterial, antiviral, anticancer, and is an excellent natural antibiotic to prevent and treat infection. We recommend odorless (deodorized or coated) garlic capsules, which contain 350 mg each. These products seem to be just as effective as the fresh, aromatic form.

N-acetylcysteine (NAC):

This is an amino acid and antioxidant that enhances the power of vitamin C and is needed to produce glutathione, the antioxidant enzyme. It also helps the liver do its job of detoxifying medications and is traditionally used to reduce mucus.

ACTION STEP:

SUPPLEMENTS FOR RELIEF OF SYMPTOMS

Nutritional supplements work primarily as preventers; however, in some cases, an extra amount of certain nutrients may be taken when symptoms of asthma, cold or flu, or allergies occur. The following amounts are the total amount to be taken, and include the optimum amounts your child is already taking daily. Administer until symptoms are relieved. Dosages are for children ages 6-12; see pages 137 and 138 for guidelines on other age groups.

For Asthma Symptoms:

At the first sign of asthma symptoms, give your child the following:

- Vitamin C: 500 mg per hour, or to bowel tolerance (see box).
- Vitamin B-6: 50 to 100 mg daily in divided doses.
- Magnesium: 300 to 400 mg per day. Magnesium is also an effective preventer of nighttime bronchial spasms. In addition, we recommend 100 to 150 mg, preferably in liquid form, before bedtime in children who are prone to nighttime flare-ups.

For Allergy Symptoms:

At the first sign of allergy symptoms, or beginning the day before you predict exposure to allergens, give your child the following:

- Vitamin C: 500 mg every hour or to bowel tolerance (see box).

- Quercetin: 300 mg twice a day.
- Pantothenic acid: 1,000 mg in divided doses

For Cold and Flu Symptoms

At the first sign of a cold or flu, give your child the following supplements:

- Vitamin C: 500 mg four times a day, or to bowel tolerance (see box).
- Beta-carotene: 25,000 IU daily, in divided doses.
- Garlic: 1–3 odorless capsules a day in divided doses.
- Zinc: 1 lozenge every two hours, up to four times a day.

HOW MUCH VITAMIN C?

When determining the optimum dosage for vitamin C, we often employ the "bowel tolerance" method, especially during crises such as colds, flu, allergic reactions, and asthma episodes. This is based on the observation that when you are sick, your body can absorb and utilize much more vitamin C than when you are well, and that your body will let you know how much you need through a phenomenon called "bowel tolerance." Here's how it works: The first time you give your child large doses of vitamin C while sick, start with 1 or 2 grams a day. Then add one gram each day until you notice symptoms of gas, bloating, or diarrhea. Then cut back down on the dosage so that bowel symptoms disappear. Be sure to divide the doses over the course of the day. For example, if you are giving 1,500 milligrams, give 500 milligrams with each meal. After symptoms have abated, be sure to taper off gradually, so the body has a chance to adjust. We recommend you use the powdered ascorbate form because it is more easily absorbed and it is easier to control the dosage.

ACTION STEP:

WORKING WITH A NUTRITION PROFESSIONAL

If your child does not seem to improve with the Optimum Daily Amounts of nutrients we have suggested here, consider working with a nutrition specialist. Make sure he or she has at least a master's degree in nutrition and has experience working with high doses of nutrients in children. When you work with a knowledgeable professional, you will get a more individualized program that takes into consideration any other conditions your child may have, and any other special needs. If needed, you will be guided in using higher amounts than we can safely recommend in a book without clinical supervision and monitoring. In our practice, we have gotten superb results with higher levels of certain nutrients such as magnesium. In addition, if you consult with a nutritionally oriented physician, your child will be able to receive intravenous injections of certain nutrients he or she may need.

The healthy food and nutritional supplements recommended in this chapter and in Chapter 6 work hand in hand and can go a long way in controlling your child's asthma. However, most children need the extra boost that medicinal herbs provide. In the next chapter, we share with you the herbs that we most often prescribe that we have found help take children to the next level of asthma control.

EIGHT   **HERBS AND OTHER
                         <u>PLANT REMEDIES</u>**

Herbal medicine is one of the oldest healing systems worldwide. While we Americans may think nothing of taking an
aspirin to ease a headache, millions of other people think nothing
of taking a few cups of willow bark tea to accomplish the same
thing. Herbs were the original medicines and are still powerful
healers. They are a crucial component of our Natural Asthma
Control Program because many herbs have specific actions that
can benefit children with asthma in several ways. Herbs may—and
often do—work more slowly than conventional drugs, but they are
also more gentle. They urge the body towards healing, and compared with drugs are virtually risk free.

In this chapter, you'll learn about the herbs we most frequently recommend in our practice to prevent flare-ups or to
reduce and alleviate symptoms when they occur. We also include
herbs that help prevent and treat allergies and upper respiratory
infections which can trigger asthma flare-ups. We first explain the
basic principles of herbal therapy. We then help you determine
the herb or herbs most suited to your child's needs and show you
how you can use herbs on your own at home. Then we describe
what you can expect when you go to a professional herbalist. We
end the chapter with a section on homeopathy, which uses many
remedies that are derived from herbs and plants.

When you integrate herbs into your Natural Asthma Control

Program, you will have plenty of company. According to Rob McCaleb, president of the Herb Research Foundation, there are over eighteen hundred herbs sold in the United States today. In 1997, Americans spent an estimated $3.2 billion on herbs.

> **REMINDER:** When you take any of the steps in this chapter, remember to continue your child's regular medical treatment. Do not reduce asthma medications on your own—do this only under the advice and supervision of your child's physician. If your child shows any of the danger signs of an asthma flare-up (see page 59, Chapter 4), seek medical attention immediately.

HERB BASICS

Technically, *herbs* refers to the above-ground parts of plants, but we and other progressive practitioners use this term to include all parts of the plants as well as certain medicinal mushrooms. Herbs are called "nature's pharmacy" and have been used for thousands of years to treat many disorders. Before the advent of synthetic drugs, all civilizations relied on the healing properties of plants. You may be surprised to learn that even today, herbs are the basis of about half of the drugs used in conventional Western medicine. For example, digitalis is made from foxglove, and aspirin was originally made from the white willow.

Although much of our knowledge of herbs comes from tradition and folk medicine, herbs have also been studied scientifically. Germany, for example, has set up a special agency devoted to evaluating herbs using the same methods and standards used to evaluate drugs. Today, about 70 percent of doctors in Germany consistently prescribe herbal medicines. Herbs are the centerpiece of many Eastern medicine systems, which are becoming more accepted in the West. Today many formerly exotic herbs are increasingly available in this country, particularly herbal formulas that have withstood the test of time.

Buying and Using Herbs Wisely

Although they work in a similar way as conventional drugs—by their biochemical effect—herbal remedies are generally gentler and safer. In contrast to conventional medicine, rather than isolating a single active agent, herbal therapy uses the whole plant or whole parts of the plant such as leaves, flowers, or roots. This can increase their effectiveness, while decreasing the side effects that may occur when using isolated components. That's why, in any form, herbs are well suited to the sensitive bodies of babies and children. However, just because herbs are "natural" doesn't mean they never have any detrimental effects. Like pharmaceuticals, you should use herbs cautiously and wisely.

In the United States, virtually all herbs are in regulatory limbo—these medicines are not officially approved by the Food and Drug Administration, and therefore there is no government agency to oversee their purity and potency. There have been reports of herb products contaminated with harmful substances such as heavy metals, and of Chinese herbal products that contain drugs among their many ingredients. We want to assure you that we have been using herbs in our clinics for fifteen years, including several Chinese herbal formulas. We have never had a problem with toxicity and are confident that reports of problems are isolated and relatively rare, especially when you compare them with all of the thousands of adverse effects from conventional drugs reported each year.

Still, as a parent, safety is paramount. Therefore, we advise you to read labels carefully. Avoid buying herbal formulas that have not been specifically recommended by a knowledgeable health practitioner, particularly those formulated in China or Hong Kong, since many of the reported problems of contamination and adulteration with drugs have been with products made in those countries. And when buying any herb or herbal formula, be sure to buy from well-established, reputable companies.

What Form to Use?

The Food and Drug Administration does not regulate herbs because the agency considers herbs to be foods, not drugs. Indeed, sometimes the line between medicinal herb and food has been blurry—our ancestors surely ate some plants that today we classify as herbs. In modern times, we still use small amounts of spices and herbs in cooking and in herbal teas, and some herbalists advocate buying whole dried herbs and preparing your own tinctures, extracts, and infusions. But to achieve the greatest accuracy, consistency, and predictability of effectiveness, we generally recommend medicinal herbs in commercially prepared, concentrated, premeasured liquids and pills. Most busy parents also prefer the convenience of commercially prepared herbs in liquid (tincture or extract) or pill form (tablets or capsules). In the "Resources" section of this book we have included a selection of herb suppliers with a reputation for high-quality products.

You can buy and use herbs individually, or you can buy and use them in combination. Combination herbal formulas are available ready-made, or you can mix them yourself from individual tinctures and extracts. We prefer organically grown herbs to reduce the risk of using herbs contaminated with pesticides.

Liquid Tinctures and Extracts.

These are concentrated liquid preparations of whole herbs or their known active constituents. They are traditionally preserved in alcohol. Tinctures and extracts last almost indefinitely if stored in a cool, dark place. In young children, liquid herbs are more easily administered than pills, and the dosage is easier to control, since they are measured by drops.

Some children object to the taste, but you can disguise the taste of tinctures and extracts by mixing them with fruit or vegetable juices. Sometimes, kids aren't fooled by this tactic, and manage not to finish the juice, leaving parents in the dark about how much of the herb their child actually swallowed. In these cases, it's better to be firm and get it over with by giving your child the herb straight or mixed with a little water, telling child, "down the hatch." If you start your child on herbs when he is very young, taste may not be a problem; as one mother tells us, "Tommy was raised on echinacea, so he's used to the taste by now."

Parents sometimes tell us they are concerned about the alcohol and wish to avoid it. Fortunately, some manufacturers, such as Herbs for Kids, use glycerin, a carbohydrate. In addition, glycerin has a naturally sweet flavor that is more palatable for children than alcohol-based tinctures and extracts.

Capsules or Tablets.

Pills are made from the whole herb or from an extract. It can be difficult to get young children to take pills, and unless you are treating an older teenager who can take the adult dosage, it may be difficult to divide a pill or capsule to obtain the appropriate amount. If you wish, you can open up a capsule or crush a pill and mix all or part of it with soft food such as applesauce to disguise the taste.

NOTE: The herbs recommended in this chapter are generally regarded as safe for children at the doses recommended. Occasionally a child may be sensitive or allergic to a particular herb. To be safe, do a sensitivity test when he or she is not having symptoms. Give your child a small amount (about half the recommended dosage), then wait for two hours. If you notice any unusual reaction, do not use that herb. The most common symptoms of herb intolerance are nausea, vomiting, diarrhea, or allergic reactions; however, these are rare and extremely variable depending on both the herb and the individual.

Most side effects from herbs are idiosyncratic—they vary unpredictably from person to person. If you notice any questionable reaction, discontinue the herb(s) at once. If your reaction is severe, call your local Poison Control Center and go to the emergency room of the nearest hospital.

Using Herbs to Prevent and Treat Asthma

There is no single "antiasthma" herb. Rather, herbs are used to prevent and treat asthma because of their various functions, which include the ability to reduce inflammation, to dilate the bronchioles, to help the body detoxify, and to enhance normal immune function. Herbs useful for prevention are also used to treat symptoms when they occur—for example, echinacea or lobelia—but they are administered more often and for a shorter duration.

What follows is our selection of the herbs that are most commonly used because they are the most effective in the greatest number of people. You may want to use herbs individually, at least at first. Using single herbs helps you determine which specific herbs work best for your child and reduces the chance of an adverse reaction. However, herbs are ultimately more effective when used in combination. You may use one of the commercial herbal formulas available, or make your own using the herbs we recommend.

DOSAGE GUIDELINES

We recommend that you buy a product that includes dosage levels for children, if possible, and follow the directions on the label. Potencies do vary and it is not always appropriate to simply divide the adult dosage down and give it to a child. However, if you cannot find a product with children's dosages, use the following as a guide. Remember, if a little is good, more is not necessarily better. If you have any doubts about dosage, consult a qualified herbalist. We do not recommend home use of herbs in babies under six months of age. Herbs are usually administered three times a day for prevention and every two to four hours for symptom relief.

The following refers to tinctures and extracts of individual or combination formulas. These are the dosages we generally recommend:

- for children aged 12 and up and 57" tall or more—20 drops of tincture or extract (or the adult dosage)
- for children aged 6–12 and 45" to 57" tall—10 drops of tincture or extract (or half the adult dosage)
- for children aged 2–6 and 34" to 45" in height—5 drops of tincture or extract 1/4 the adult dosage)
- for children ages 1–2, consult with a nutritional professional

Commercial Herbal Formulas.

There are several combination remedies formulated for use in asthma, colds and flu, and allergies. Like our patients, you may get good results with them, but will probably need to experiment to see which is most effective in your child. If you don't notice any improvement, try another herb or a combination formula. If that doesn't work, then move on to another herb or try a different combination.

Chinese Herbal Formulas.

Chinese herbs are prescribed according to very different criteria than are Western herbs, although a growing number of Chinese herbs are also used by Western herbalists. These include astragalus, ma huang (ephedra), and licorice. To give you a glimpse of the way Chinese herbs are prescribed, consider, for example, the two formulas we use regularly in our health centers, with great success, to strengthen the lungs, boost immunity, reduce inflammation, and relax the airways. As a general tonic and preventive, we use "Strengthen Lung," which replenishes lung moisture, expels mucus, relaxes the chest, regulates qi (the vital force), and wards off excess "wind, heat, and cold." When a child has frequent infections that precipitate asthma flare-ups, we use "Purge External Wind," which increases resistance to "external wind," believed to be the major force in the development of illness, and paves the way for other disease-bearers such as "cold" and "dampness." There are also patent remedies for specific conditions such as colds and flu that are available without a prescription in health food stores and Chinese pharmacies. Again, we recommend that for safety's sake, avoid those manufactured in Hong Kong.

Making and Using Herbal Formulas

It's a very simple process to make your own herbal formulas, and it allows you to tailor the formula to your child's needs and responses. Simply buy herbs in tincture or extract form, empty the entire contents of each container into a larger glass container, and mix well. Refill the original containers with the formula and relabel them, including the date. Use the dosages provided in the dosage guidelines on page 155. It's generally best to give your child herbs along with his meals. At the end of this chapter, we provide a glossary of the herbs we recommend.

HERBS FOR PREVENTION

These are our favorite herbal formulas. Use one or more of them, depending on your child's needs. Unless otherwise noted, combine equal amounts of each of the herbs listed for each formula. Administer each formula two to three times a day for one month, then assess your child's condition according to the guidelines we provide in Chapter 4.

Basic Asthma Prevention Formula

The following Basic Prevention Formula is the most effective all-round preventer of asthma flare-ups as well as colds, flu, and allergies which can trigger flare-ups. If you give your child only one formula, this should be it.

- Astragalus
- Echinacea
- Milk thistle
- Green tea
- Grindelia
- Hops or Valerian
- Coleus forskohlii
- Ginkgo biloba
- Picrorhiza kurroa
- Licorice
- Feverfew
- Lobelia (use half the amount of other herbs)

Immune System Strengtheners

If your child is particularly prone to upper respiratory infections, which can trigger asthma, he may benefit from the following formula.

- Astragalus
- Echinacea
- Shiitake or maitake mushroom
- Goldenseal (do not use for a prolonged period of time)
- Cleavers

ACTION STEP:

HERBS FOR RELIEF OF ASTHMA SYMPTOMS

When your child is beginning to show signs of asthma symptoms, use the following formula, which contains the most effective commonly used herbs. Administer every two to four hours until symptoms subside. If you prefer, you may use lobelia alone every fifteen minutes during an acute asthma flare-up.

- Lobelia (use half the amount of other herbs)
- Ephedra
- Licorice
- Green tea
- Grindelia
- St. John's wort
- Valerian

ACTION STEP:

HERBS FOR RELIEF OF ALLERGY SYMPTOMS

Allergic reactions to airborne allergens such as pollen, house dust, and animal dander can trigger asthma. Herbs can reduce these allergic symptoms without suppressing them. During an allergic reaction, administer the following herbal formula every two to four hours, until symptoms subside.

- Nettles
- Licorice
- Angelica

For eczema:

Asthmatic children often also suffer from eczema, an inflammatory allergic skin condition that, if suppressed with cortisone cream, can drive the condition deeper and worsen asthma. If your child experiences eczema, add burdock and red clover to the above herbal formula. You may use natural ointments or creams that contain licorice or German chamomile. In one study, licorice was found to be more effective than cortisone (93 percent improvement versus 83 percent.).

ACTION STEP:

HERBS FOR RELIEF OF COLD AND FLU SYMPTOMS

During a cold or flu, the following formula may help boost your child's immune system and break up congestion. Administer every two to four hours, until symptoms subside.

- Echinacea
- Goldenseal (do not use for a prolonged period of time)
- Ephedra

If there is cough and congested lungs, add one or more of the following to the above formula:

- Mullein
- Horehound
- Red clover

You may also want to try a commercial herb-based cough medicine. These tend to be gentler than the conventional variety. As the parent of an asthmatic boy said to us, "My son sometimes developed a terrible cough—it sounded like a harsh bark and continued for twenty-four hours. In desperation I would give him cough medicine, but it would dry him up so much, and I knew that was bad for his asthma. I knew we wanted him to have a productive cough because if the airways get too dry, they become clogged and irritated and that can trigger an asthma flare-up."

GLOSSARY OF HERBS

- *Angelica*. This is a traditional Chinese and Japanese herb used to prevent and treat allergies to pollen, house dust, and animals. It appears to inhibit allergy-related antibodies.

- *Astragalus*. A potent immune system strengthener that enhances interferon production, astragalus is a traditional Chinese herb that is generally used as a preventive tonic for general disease resistance and increased energy. It is considered to specifically strengthen and tone the lungs. Studies from China have demonstrated that astragalus may both lower the incidence of colds as well as shorten their duration and lessen their severity.

- *Cleavers.* Also known as clivers or goose grass, cleavers has many traditional uses. It is favored for its ability to restore an inflamed, swollen lymphatic system, and may therefore calm the chronic inflammation that is the underlying cause of asthma.

- *Coleus forskohlii.* This is an herb traditionally used in Ayurveda (traditional East Indian) medicine for asthma, allergies, and inflammatory skin conditions such as eczema. There is extensive research to support these uses, as it has been proven to stimulate biochemical reactions that cause smooth muscles to relax and, hence, ease breathing. It is most widely available under the trade name Forskolin.

- *Echinacea.* Research shows that echinacea is the premier immune-boosting tonic herb. Echinacea appears to work by increasing levels of interferon, an antiviral substance produced by the body, stimulating white cell production, and through its immune-boosting and anti-inflammatory constituents called polysaccharides. Echinacea will cause your child's tongue to tingle for a few minutes after taking it; this is not dangerous—it is a sign that the preparation is potent. As an immune booster/preventive, some herbalists recommend that this herb be taken for eight weeks with a break for one week before resuming, but others, such as ourselves, feel it is advisable to take it daily.

PRECAUTIONS: Echinacea is safe for most people but shouldn't be taken during pregnancy or by people with tuberculosis or diseases thought to have an autoimmune component, such as lupus and multiple sclerosis.

- *Elecampane.* Also known as horseheal, elecampane has been used in many cultures for centuries to treat many types of respiratory problems. It encourages expectoration and therefore is especially useful when your child has a cough.

- *Ephedra or Ma huang.* Ma huang is the name of an herb used in Chinese medicine that contains a natural form of ephedrine, which is the chemical included in larger amounts in asthma medications such as Tedral. Ephedrine affects the body similar to adrenaline—it stimulates the nervous system, reduces swelling in the mucus membranes of the nose and sinuses, and dilates the bronchial tubes. According to a 1985 study, ephedrine's anti-inflammatory action takes place at the early stage of inflammation, and this inhibits the formation of the inflammatory chemical prostaglandins. Ephedra is included in many commercial combination remedies for asthma and upper respiratory infections. Ephedra can also break up congestion due to hay fever.

  PRECAUTIONS: Overuse of this herb can increase heart rate and blood pressure and result in anxiety and insomnia. Long-term use can eventually tax the adrenal gland. Some states have limited the amount of ephedra that a product can contain.

- *Feverfew.* A traditional herb used for a variety of conditions, feverfew, a member of the chrysanthemum family, has recently been shown to inhibit histamine and other inflammatory chemicals.

- *Ginkgo biloba.* Gingko is a potent anti-inflammatory herb that may ease inflammation, asthma, and allergies. A famous Chinese herb traditionally used for allergies, this herb has been extensively studied in Europe and has recently become popular in the United States because it improves blood circulation, including blood flow to the brain. It appears that ginkgo dampens platelet-activating factor (PAF), which is part of the inflammatory cascade. Clinical research indicates that you need to take ginkgo for at least twelve weeks before you see results, although many people report results in two to three weeks.

- *Goldenseal.* As a general tonic, goldenseal is often used to treat chronic conditions involving the production of mucus. It is especially useful when combined with coltsfoot in treating chronic coughs. However, you should not give goldenseal to your child indefinitely.

- *Green tea (Camellia sinesis).* There are many studies demonstrating that green tea is a potent antioxidant.

- *Grindelia camporum.* This herb is traditionally used in asthma because of its antispasmotic properties.

- *Horehound.* Horehound is a good herb to have handy for a bad cough due to colds or bronchitis. A potent expectorant, it helps clear away mucus in the chest.

- *Licorice.* Licorice is a general tonic that particularly stimulates health in the chest, loosens mucus, and helps purify the blood. Licorice is often combined with other herbs to consolidate and energize them and thus is a component of many herbal formulas. In addition to strengthening the lungs, licorice is a potent anti-inflammatory that dampens allergic reactions. It inhibits the enzyme needed to produce the inflammatory chemicals prostaglandins and leukotrienes.

PRECAUTIONS: Licorice is generally a safe herb, but may raise blood pressure and therefore should not be taken by anyone with a history of hypertension, diabetes, glaucoma, stroke, or heart disease, or who is pregnant or nursing.

- *Lobelia*. Also called "asthma weed," lobelia is traditionally used in many cultures to strengthen the lungs and prevent asthma. Lobelia appears to stimulate the adrenal gland to produce hormones that relax the bronchial muscles. It also acts as an expectorant, loosening mucus so your child can cough it up more effectively, clearing the air passages.

- *Milk Thistle*. This herb is very popular in Europe, where several studies have shown it to enhance liver function. In fact, German health officials recognize milk thistle as helpful in treating many disorders of the liver. It contains a chemical called silymarin which helps regenerate liver cells and purify the liver of toxins.

- *Mullein*. This herb is known to be a good expectorant and helps clear the chest of mucus as well as soothes an irritated throat and bronchial passages.

- *Nettles*. This herb has been used in many cultures around the world to treat nasal and respiratory problems including allergies, coughs, and chest congestion. In a double-blind study of sixty-nine people with allergies, nearly 50 percent found stinging nettles to be as effective as their conventional antihistamine medication, according to study results published in 1990.

- *Picrorhiza kurroa*. Many studies of this herb, traditionally used in Indian medicine, show that it inhibits the release of histamine and has many other effects that benefit asthmatics. This is not a common herb, but it's available at large health food stores and by mail from the companies listed in "Resources."

- *Red clover*. This herb is known for its immune-enhancing ability and for its antispasmodic and expectorant properties. It thus is often recommended for coughs due to congested mucus and as a treatment for skin inflammations such as eczema.

- *Shiitake or maitake mushroom*. These mushrooms have been extensively used in Asia for thousands of years and their immune-enhancing abilities are now being confirmed through scientific study. Recent studies of shiitake extract, for example, have shown it to have antitumor, antiviral, and immune-stimulating effects as well as other benefits.

- *St. John's wort*. Relaxes and soothes nerves; it also relaxes muscles, including the bronchial muscles, and therefore eases breathing.

- *Valerian*. This has a long tradition as a calming herb so it may prevent stress-related asthma; it relaxes muscle spasms and cramps and may be useful as a bronchodilator.

ACTION STEP:

SEEING A PROFESSIONAL HERBALIST

If you do not get the results you want using herbs for self-care at home, consider working with a professional herbalist or medical doctor who specializes in herbs and other natural therapies. An herbalist will not only be able to guide you in using herbs to treat the acute symptoms but to treat the underlying condition that leads to asthma flare-ups as well. During a visit with an herbalist, expect to be evaluated physically, emotionally, and mentally. As a natural health practitioner, the herbalist will spend whatever time is needed to determine the imbalance and disharmony that is at the root of your condition.

Unfortunately, there is no certification or licensing process in this country specifically for herbalists. However, herbal medicine is used by many licensed medical doctors (M.D.'s), nurse practitioners (L.N.P.'s), naturopathic physicians (N.D.'s), and acupuncturists. To find one of these health professionals who is licensed to practice in your state, ask for referrals from friends who are under the care of an herbalist, or inquire about local herbalists at your health food store. You may also contact the organizations in the "Resources" section of this book for referral to a knowledgeable herbalist in your geographic area.

Once you have the names of one or more herbalists, call each of their offices and ask where he or she studied herbalism and how long the herbalist has been practicing. The School of Medical Herbalism and its affiliates have an excellent reputation for producing well-trained herbalists. You may also ask the herbalist for the names of patients he or she has treated or is treating now.

HOMEOPATHY

Homeopathy was developed in the late 1700s by a German physician named Samuel Hahnemann. He developed this gentle medicine as a reaction to the harsh methods of dealing with sickness in the eighteenth century, which included bloodletting and purging. Today, homeopathy is the fastest-growing medicine in the world and is also growing in popularity in the United States.

Since its inception, homeopathy has been used to treat a wide variety of illnesses, including asthma. There is also a growing body of scientific evidence that homeopathy works for many complaints, including asthma. For example, there are three studies that show homeopathy improves allergic asthma. The latest was published in December 1994 in Britain's leading medical journal,

The Lancet. This double-blind, placebo-controlled study compared homeopathy against a placebo (dummy medicine). Only five out of thirteen patients receiving the placebo improved, but nine out of eleven patients receiving homeopathy improved, and their improvement was more pronounced and longer lasting (eight weeks). In the hands of a skilled homeopath, the aim of this form of therapy is often to cure the underlying disease and prevent flare-ups. This goal is beyond home care homeopathy.

In our clinics, we sometimes work with parents who use homeopathic remedies. Homeopathy considers asthma to be a deep-seated condition that requires professional homeopathic treatment to cure. This is beyond the scope of our book. However, you may want to try homeopathy in your home to safely and effectively relieve symptoms of an asthma flare-up and to treat allergic reactions and upper respiratory infections that often trigger or worsen asthmatic episodes.

If you would like to consult with a professional homeopath, see the "Resources" section of this book for sources for directories of homeopaths.

Understanding Homeopathy

Homeopathy uses infinitesimal amounts of substances derived mainly from plants; some remedies also come from minerals or animals. Remedies are based on the principle that "like cures like," which grew out of the time-honored observation that substances that cause harmful symptoms in healthy people can, in very diluted doses, cure similar symptoms in sick people. So, for example, if your child has a cold with runny nose and burning, watery eyes, she may benefit from a homeopathic remedy called allium cepa, which is made from onion.

As with other forms of natural medicine, according to homeopathy, symptoms are signs that your body is trying to deal with an underlying disorder or imbalance, and therefore should not be suppressed. Taking a remedy that matches the symptoms of your illness stimulates and supports your symptoms and strengthens your body's innate healing power, part of your "vital force." Eventually your body no longer needs the symptoms and they fade away naturally.

In using homeopathy at home, you could be helping your child's asthma in several ways. By giving your child homeopathic medicines instead of conventional medicines to treat immediate symptoms of allergies, infections, and asthma, you reduce the toxic burden and hence avoid worsening the underlying condition and driving it deeper. You also help lessen the chance that allergies and infections will trigger the asthma. And by working *with* your child's immune system, not against it, you can help normalize and strengthen your child's immune system, rather than weaken it. There are also many homeopathic remedies for childhood illnesses including colic, teething difficulties, earache, bed-wetting, measles, mumps, and chicken pox. You may also treat stress homeopathically. By treating as many ailments as possible with homeopathy you also avoid adding to your child's toxic load.

The Basics of Homeopathic Home Care

Homeopathic remedies come in several forms: small tablets or pellets that contain a tiny amount of sugar and liquids that contain tiny amounts of alcohol. Homeopathic remedies are available in health food stores, pharmacies, and through the mail as single remedies and combination remedies.

We recommend you first try single remedies because they are more personalized and more potent than combination remedies. However, prescribing them correctly requires more effort. That's why many people begin with the combination remedies that are becoming popular (see below). There are about two hundred to three hundred commonly used single remedies, each with their own symptom pattern. To be most effective, you need to choose a remedy carefully to get the best match. In this chapter are brief descriptions of symptom patterns for the most commonly used remedies for acute asthma episodes, colds and flu, and allergies. We have been necessarily brief in our descriptions of the full symptom patterns. If none of the single remedies suggested below is effective, refer to one of the books devoted entirely to homeopathy listed in the "Resources" section of this book, or try a combination remedy.

How to Administer Homeopathic Remedies

Homeopathy follows its own rules of administration:

- Potency: Use 12x, 12c, 30x, or 30c potency.

- Dosage: Follow the dosage amounts on the product label for children; generally 1–2 pills or 5–10 drops is one dose.

- Frequency and duration: The frequency of the dosage depends on the intensity of the symptoms; the more severe the symptoms, the more frequent the dose. You increase the potency by taking the same small dose more frequently—taking more pellets or drops per dose won't increase the potency. The first day symptoms occur, administer the remedy every one or two hours for up to six doses. Beginning the next day, administer three times daily for up to a further five days.

- When to stop: Always stop if you see improvement and repeat only if the remedy helped and the same symptoms return. Try another remedy if there is no improvement after the first three doses. If there is no improvement whatsoever after the first three doses, you have probably chosen the wrong remedy. Move down the list of recommended remedies and choose the next one that best fits your case and repeat the dosing process. If the second remedy is not working, you may want to try a third.

To give homeopathy the best chance of working, it's best to follow these guidelines:

- Avoid touching the remedy with your hands, or your child touching it. Rather, tip the required number of pellets into the container cap and then into your child's mouth; if tablets are blister-packed, pop them directly into your child's mouth. Touching the remedy could contaminate or inactivate it.

- Instruct your child to let the remedy dissolve slowly under the tongue so it is absorbed directly through the inner surfaces of the mouth (mucosa). Some combination tablets instruct you to chew them instead. The remedy is absorbed into the bloodstream, and thus acts very quickly.

- Giving an infant or very young child a homeopathic remedy can be tricky. It's not necessary that the child swallow it, as long as it touches the inner surfaces of the mouth. If you are giving an infant a liquid remedy, one or two drops should suffice. If you are using pellets or tablets, you may want to crush one between two pieces of clean paper so it will dissolve more quickly.

- Your child should avoid eating or drinking anything except filtered water for fifteen minutes to a half hour before and after taking the remedy.

• • •

Store homeopathic remedies in the original container, away from heat, sunlight, and strong-smelling substances that might contaminate them; the list includes perfumes, camphor, and eucalyptus (found in many cosmetics and other common medicine cabinet items such as Tiger balm, Vicks products, and lip balms).

Choosing a Remedy

Homeopathy is unique in taking into account the emotional and psychological characteristics of the patient. There is not one universal remedy for asthma because people differ from one another, and so do their asthma symptoms.

Combination homeopathic remedies are an excellent alternative to single remedies and are more user-friendly for beginners. They are specifically labeled for "asthma," "colds," "flu," and "allergies," as well as specific symptoms such as "sore throat" or "cough." Combination products contain two or more of the single remedies that are most often used to treat that symptom or condition. Therefore, this "shotgun" approach increases the chance that a product will contain the remedy you need, but at a low potency.

If you don't get relief from a particular remedy or combination remedy, don't give up on homeopathy. Try another remedy or brand until you find the right "fit." You may need to consult a homeopathic physician for help in finding the right remedy.

ACTION STEP:

HOMEOPATHIC REMEDIES FOR RELIEF OF ASTHMA SYMPTOMS

When your child is beginning to show signs of asthma symptoms, choose among the following most commonly used remedies to treat mild to moderate symptoms during an acute episode.

Administer as instructed above. If your child does not respond to homeopathy, or suffers from severe symptoms, use the conventional medicine outlined in your treatment plan. Make sure your child drinks plenty of liquids to replace the water lost by rapid breathing and to keep mucus liquid and loose.

- *Arsenicum:* This is the most useful remedy for this condition. Use this when your child is markedly fearful, restless, and weak; if your child has symptoms of hay fever or coughing; if symptoms get worse between midnight and 3 A.M. Children who benefit from arsenicum are usually chilly and feel better when they are warm. They tend to be thirsty and like frequent sips of water.

- *Pulsatilla:* This is the remedy to use when there is a lot of mucus in the chest that causes coughing, when wheezing begins or is worse in the evening and at night, and symptoms are worse after eating. Children who benefit from pulsatilla are sweet, affectionate, tearful, and clingy; they usually feel oppressed by warm, stuffy rooms and aren't thirsty.

- *Ipecac:* Use this remedy for asthma that is characterized by a lot of phlegm in the chest, wheezing, and coughing that arrives in intense spasms; the child may be nauseous and coughing may bring on vomiting. Children who are helped by ipecac look pale, sickly, and exhausted. The symptoms are similar to pulsatilla, but the child does not have the personality traits of that remedy, and there is even more mucus.

- *Spongia:* This is the remedy when there is raspy breathing with wheezing, but little or no mucus; if the symptoms began after being chilled or triggered by a cold; if wheezing began suddenly and worsens during sleep; if your child has a dry cough that sounds like a bark. Try this remedy if your child becomes short of breath when lying down or with movement, but improves when he tips his head back or if he feels better when you give him warm foods or beverages.

• *Sambucus:* The symptoms are similar to arsenicum, but the child doesn't have the personality traits of that remedy—less fear and restlessness. The child may feel she is suffocating and symptoms get worse after midnight. If arsenicum doesn't help, try this one.

• *Lobelia:* For wheezing and feeling of tightness in the chest, when symptoms begin after the child gets chilled, and breathing cold air makes the episode worse. Unlike spongia, the breathing isn't noisy. The child may tend to feel somewhat better around noon.

• *Blatta Orientalis:* For asthma that is associated with bronchitis, when your child is very congested and has a lot of pus-like mucus, and when the likely trigger is household dust, especially when it may contain cockroach allergens.

ACTION STEP:

HOMEOPATHIC REMEDIES FOR RELIEF OF ALLERGY SYMPTOMS

Allergies, eczema, and asthma are part of the allergic condition known as atopy. Although hay fever is a trigger, and eczema can drive a child frantic with itching, neither should be suppressed because this can drive the asthma deeper. Treating these allergic conditions homeopathically eases symptoms without suppressing them and thus may indirectly help your child's asthma.

Allergies to Airborne Allergens

• *Allium cepa:* If symptoms include a profuse, watery, burning discharge from the nose; frequent sneezing; a red and sore nose; and watery eyes that are sore and burn. Allium is particularly indicated when the person sneezes upon entering a warm room. Possible accompanying symptoms include headache, cough, and hoarseness—all of which improve in the open air.

• *Euphrasia:* When most of the symptoms affect the eyes, which tear, swell, burn, and are sensitive to light. The discharge from the eye is irritating to the skin but nasal discharge is bland and sneezing does not occur in violent bouts. Symptoms are worse in the evening, in light, and indoors.

• *Pulsatilla:* When the eyes produce a sticky, thick, yellow discharge and eyes are itchy and burn, there is copious tearing, and eyes feel worse with warmth.

• *Eczema graphites:* When the eczema is "wet" and exudes a fluid resembling honey, especially if it occurs in the flexion points (such as elbows) or on the palms of the hands, between toes, and around the genitals and mouth; symptoms worsen with warmth and around menstruation; they improve with cold applications.

• *Petroleum:* For dry, scaly eczema that appears during cold weather or wintertime. Symptoms are worse in winter and with damp and cold; they are better in summer and with dry warmth.

• *Sulfur:* For dry, scaly, itchy, burning eczema of the scalp; symptoms are worse with scratching or moist warmth such as bathing and better with dry warmth.

• *Ointments:* There are several ointments available to treat eczema, including graphites and calendula ointments. Boericke & Tafel make a cream called Florasone containing a medicinal tropical vine that has been shown in three studies to effectively relieve symptoms of eczema.

ACTION STEP:

HOMEOPATHIC REMEDIES FOR RELIEF OF COLD AND FLU SYMPTOMS

An upper respiratory tract infection often precipitates an asthma attack. Homeopathy offers real help in terms of relieving symptoms of a current infection, as well strengthening the body's response to future infections. In fact, evidence suggests that homeopathy was more effective than conventional therapy during the great flu epidemics of the early 1900s. The following are the most popular single remedies used for colds and flu.

• *Aconite:* This remedy is sometimes called the vitamin C of homeopathy because it is most effective during the early stage of a cold, especially when the cold symptoms appear suddenly and violently after exposure to cold weather or wind; when there is a clear, watery runny nose and a lot of sneezing; if your child has a red, hot, dry sore throat; fever; and coughing. Children who benefit from aconite can be restless and anxious.

• *Allium cepa:* Use this remedy when the cold symptoms include a runny nose and eyes, which may be irritating and cause burning and redness (but not under the eyes); if the larynx tickles and there is a dry, painful cough; if symptoms are worse indoors, with warmth, and in the evening, but better in the open air.

• *Pulsatilla:* This is very useful for colds that have mainly nasal symptoms; if there is thick, yellow or yellow-green, nonirritating mucus that smells bad and alternates with a thinner discharge; if your child's nose runs in fresh air and in the morning and becomes stuffy indoors and at night.

• *Mercurius:* Use this for colds or flu that bring on a painful sore throat accompanied by fever; if the throat is red and swollen and the tonsils or throat have white or yellow deposits of pus. Children who benefit from mercurius are extremely sensitive to changes in temperature and easily become chilled or overheated; they have restless and sweaty nights and are intensely thirsty for cold drinks.

• *Oscillococcinum:* This is an all-round remedy that is best used at the very first sign of flu to relieve symptoms of fever, chills, and body aches and pains. In three studies this remedy was found to be effective for fever, shivering, and ailing due to flu. One of the studies found that in the group who took the homeopathic product, fever decreased more rapidly—in two days—than in the placebo group, and shivering disappeared by day four. The second controlled study, published in 1989 in the *British Journal of Clinical Pharmacology*, found that 66 percent more of the oscillococcinum group recovered within forty-eight hours.

NINE

LIVING WELL WITH ASTHMA

If you're like most of our patients, you'll be relieved to hear that current thinking is that asthma is not psychosomatic. Stress, anxiety, or faulty parenting are *not* the cause of asthma. However, once your child has developed asthma, there's no question that you, your child, and your entire family are uniquely stressed in ways that families with healthy children are not. Wrenching changes in lifestyle, feelings of guilt and blame, the constant fear of another episode, the overwhelmingly impossible desire to protect your child from all harm, sibling rivalry, worries about the future—these are some of the most common peaks and valleys in the roller coaster ride of emotions that living with asthma presents. Furthermore, asthma—when it is poorly controlled—can interfere with your child's school, social development, and family life and can cause a great deal of financial strain. On top of the normal stresses any family faces, it should come as no surprise that some families start to creak and even crack under the strain. Unfortunately, stress can be "toxic" in the sense that if you don't learn to manage it, it can actually worsen your child's asthma, which creates more stress, in a vicious circle.

But there's good news, too. In the first place, if you are using the therapies described earlier in our Natural Asthma Control Program to bring your child's asthma under better control, you are *already* helping to minimize the difficulties that lead to stress. But there are other, specific steps you can take as well, and since our Natural Asthma Control Program takes a holistic approach, it would not be complete without providing you with a selection of those that we have found work best.

In this chapter, therefore, we deal with the emotional aspects of asthma. We reassure you that you are not alone as you struggle with your fears and frustrations, and then we provide you with a variety of ways to cope better. We first take a look at the interplay between emotions and asthma. The first action step is a self-assessment questionnaire to help you become more aware of negative, toxic emotions. The remaining action steps are some simple ways you can detoxify your child's inner and outer emotional environment; we look at some age-specific issues as well as issues, such as overprotectiveness and fearing the worst, that can affect your family no matter what your child's age. We then help you deal with issues surrounding school and day care and conclude the chapter by discussing the issue of seeking emotional support outside the home.

There's more good news: We have seen time and time again how successfully overcoming the challenge of asthma can be a growth experience for the whole family and the child with asthma in particular. It can teach personal responsibility, develop self-discipline, and instill confidence. You, your child, and your family *can* live well with asthma—and perhaps live better because of it.

REMINDER: When you take any of the steps in this chapter, remember to continue your child's regular medical treatment. Do not reduce asthma medications on your own—do this only under the advice and supervision of your child's physician. If your child shows any of the danger signs of an asthma flare-up (see page 59, Chapter 4), seek medical attention immediately.

THE BENEFITS OF COPING BETTER

Coping better emotionally means making changes, and change can be difficult because it involves taking a look at and challenging ingrained ways of feeling, believing, and behaving. But the rewards are great. Together with the mind-body relaxation techniques provided in the following chapter, improving your coping skills can work hand in hand with the other therapies in your Natural Asthma Control Program. Since your emotions and those of the entire family affect your child's emotions, and vice versa, it's crucial that the entire family works together to resolve stressful issues. When you succeed at this, amazing things can happen. You may help prevent asthma episodes as well as reduce your child's susceptibility to infection. You may also lessen the severity and duration of symptoms if your child has an episode. Working in the emotional arena makes it less likely that one child's asthma will become the center stage around which everything else in your life revolves. It will therefore foster better overall emotional health for the entire family. And it will make following the other steps in our Natural Asthma Control Program easier because negative emotions won't be sabotaging the confidence and positive thinking required to make the effort.

EMOTIONS AND ASTHMA

Emotions can be as toxic and cumulatively damaging as exposure to pollen, pollution, and the wrong food. Emotions and family dynamics are related to asthma in two ways: they can influence it and be influenced by it. They can come *before* a flare-up and trigger or worsen your child's condition, and they can come *after* symptoms appear and be a reaction to it. Recent work in the new field of psychoneuroimmunology (PNI) shows us that there is a definite connection between emotional states, the nervous system, the hormonal system, and immune function. As a result of recent research findings, scientists working in the field of PNI routinely refer to the immune system as a circulating nervous system. So, since stress exerts its effect via signals initiated by the nervous system, we can influence the effect of stress on the body by influencing the mind and nervous system. This helps explain how stress and poor coping strategies can add to your child's toxic burden and how managing stress and improving your coping skills can reduce the toxic burden, and thus reduce symptoms.

Two Provocative Mechanisms

Although no one is exactly clear how emotions provoke asthma, we have evidence that there are two basic mechanisms at work.

Immediate Breathing Changes.

Just as is the case with exercise-induced asthma, strong emotions can cause your child to take faster and more shallow breaths (hyperventilate). This short-term phenomenon occurs in both positive and negative emotions—laughter and excitement stimulate the nervous system and can have the same effect on breathing as crying, frustration, anger, or fear. Unfortunately, if your child has asthma, the sudden influx of cold dry air causes the hypersensitive airways to go into spasm, making breathing difficult. Once your child begins to experience an asthma flare-up, he feels like he is suffocating and he feels afraid, anxious, and panicked. This creates a vicious cycle of stress, flare-up, and more stress.

Chronic Stress and Adrenal Exhaustion.

If your child cannot fully express and deal with his negative emotions, he experiences chronic stress. This can contribute to the underlying inflammatory condition, which then with other environmental or genetic factors makes your child more prone to asthma symptoms. Chronic toxic emotions lead to chronic elevations of stress-related hormones, cortisol and norepinephrine. The nervous system signals the adrenal glands to secrete these chemicals, which are antiallergy and anti-inflammatory. With chronic stress, the adrenals eventually become exhausted and are no longer able to secrete adequate amounts of these hormones. Your child is less able to handle stress, less able to relax the airways, and less able to control inflammation and allergies; and the immune system is less able to resist infection.

Emotional Fallout

The other side of the coin—and the much more common and troublesome one—is that stress and negative emotions can be a result of having the condition. Your child may be worried that she will have another attack and feel embarrassed, self-conscious, or fearful when one occurs. She may develop a poor self-image and eventually become depressed or anxious. As a parent, you may be overly fearful and protective, or feel guilty or that you are somehow to blame. Your other children might tend to act out and get into trouble, misbehaving just to get attention for themselves. These negative emotions can also become part of the cycle of stress, flare-up, stress.

TOXIC EMOTIONS IN ACTION

We've known about the stress and asthma connection for decades. In Great Britain, the asthma mortality rate rose significantly during 1940—the year they began to be heavily bombed by Germans. Apparently, the constant threat of harm and the horrific sound of bombs exploding put everyone's body in a state of near-permanent alert. In the United States, studies show that children who are exposed to distressing sounds such as gunshots or violent incidents were twice as likely to experience wheezing or use bronchodilators, according to *Newsweek*.

Calming the Mind and the Body

As a parent who cares for your child, you have the responsibility to take care of your own stress so that it doesn't spill over and affect your child. And you have the responsibility of helping your child overcome her stresses, just as it's your responsibility to give her health-building food and medication.

As you will see later in this chapter, there are ways to calm your child, yourself, and your family so that unnecessary negative emotions don't get out of hand. But first, you need to detect signs of stress and anxiety and determine if these are playing a role. The following self-assessment helps you do just that.

ACTION STEP:
SELF-ASSESSMENT QUESTIONNAIRE

Even well-adjusted families can encounter bumps in the road as they learn to adjust to living with asthma. This questionnaire is designed to help ferret out those issues we have found to crop up most often. By becoming alert to them, you are less likely to stay stuck in them; instead, you experience them, move through them, and move on.

We hope you will use this assessment as a springboard for discussion and action to help the whole family cope better. Following the assessment, you will find a summary of the techniques we have found to be most helpful in restoring a healthy family life. If you have answered "yes" to several of these questions, chances are you could benefit from some of these techniques.

- Does your child seem reluctant to admit that he is sick, take medication, monitor symptoms, or avoid triggers? (This is especially common among teens.)
- Does he say he is afraid of having an asthma flare-up?
- Does he voluntarily limit his activities for fear of triggering an episode?
- Does he panic during an episode?
- Does he have an "I can't" attitude rather then a "can do" attitude?
- Does your child seem excessively fearful?
- Are you overly anxious or fearful?
- Do you panic when your child has an asthma episode?
- Do you assume the worst during a flare-up and think, "Ohmigod he's going to die?"
- Do you show signs of overprotectiveness?
- Are you in the habit of seeing your child primarily as a sick person?
- Do you needlessly limit his activities or deny him the rights and responsibilities you would give another child his age?
- Do you grant him special privileges?
- Do you have trouble accepting that your child has asthma?
- Do you feel guilty that your child has asthma?
- Are you angry at your child's doctor?
- Do you neglect your other children and pay more attention to your child with asthma?
- Do your other children ever say they wish they had asthma too?
- Do they have behavior problems or are their grades slipping?

ACTION STEP:

GROWING UP WITH ASTHMA

Coping with asthma in infants is not the same as coping with asthma in toddlers, in school-age children, or in teenagers. You and your child will be facing different issues as she develops. Your child will also be capable of taking on different responsibilities for her care, depending on her age and maturity. As she understands asthma better and takes on greater and greater responsibility, she will feel less helpless and vulnerable and more in control. In this section, we provide you with advice on how you and your child can get through the experience of living with asthma with your psyche intact.

Infants (age one to two)

Taking care of any infant is a huge responsibility, and it's even more challenging and exhausting if your infant has asthma. It can be more frightening than asthma in an older child because you are less likely to be aware of worsening symptoms until they are quite serious. That's because your child can't tell you she is having problems early on, and because infants' lungs are so small they become clogged more easily and quickly. As a result, you may feel overly anxious and be overprotective because your child seems so small and helpless.

To ease you and your child through this period, make sure you are aware of these early warning signs in infants and monitor your child closely:

- sudden change in her sleep pattern
- green or yellow mucus in her nose
- circles under her eyes
- pale skin

- slight cough
- sudden change in behavior, such as irritability
- more drooling than usual

You might assume that a parent who has had asthma herself, and who knows the ropes, would be more relaxed around an infant with asthma. If this is not so in your case, you are not alone, according to this parent: "When you are going through an asthma flare-up yourself, you feel at least you have a tiny bit of control over it. You know what it feels like and know what you have to do. With my baby, the condition wasn't *mine*, so I felt I had less control. I was just watching on the sidelines, waiting for something to happen. It was very scary watching a two-year-old go through what I went through."

Toddlers (age three to six)

If your toddler has asthma, it is likely that your greatest concern at this stage is the effect that asthma is having on your child's burgeoning social, physical, and intellectual development. You will also be facing the task of gradually teaching your child to take on some responsibility for managing his asthma.

To help you accomplish this:

- Explain to your child, in language he will understand, what asthma is and why he is taking medication and/or natural therapies. Let him know that other children have asthma too, and that you and his doctor are going to help him breathe better.

- Ask your child periodically if there is anything he wants to know about asthma or tell you about the way he is feeling.

- Talk about asthma triggers so he can start to recognize them and avoid them.

- Teach your child the early warning signs (see Chapter 3) so he can tell you when they occur.

- Teach your child the side effects of medication so he can tell you when they occur.

- Teach your child how to use a peak flow meter, spacer, nebulizer, and, if older, an inhaler. At this stage, children can use all these things, with some assistance, and this bolsters their confidence and sense of mastery.

- Teach him to perform simple breathing exercises (in Chapter 11) and to drink water when he feels symptoms coming on.

- Have him take on household responsibilities and chores as part of his usual routine so he doesn't feel different from other children.

- Realize that he may start to refuse to go along with certain measures—such as taking herbs or pills or eating certain foods. Try to give him more choice, within reason; for example, let him choose which kind of juice you will mix with his herbal formula.

We are continually surprised at how much responsibility children can take on even at this age. The parent of one of our patients recalls, "When Ellen was just three-and-a half, she was at a kids' party at a friend's house. We had told the parents about her food allergies and restrictions, but for some reason, we forgot to mention oranges. When the adults started to give the children oranges, my daughter told them she couldn't have any because they were not good for her. I was amazed when they told me this—you don't expect a three-year-old to be that aware." Another parent says that "Even at age three, my son was able to say, 'Mommy, I have to go to the hospital *now*' when he was having a bad flare-up. By the time he had his third episode, he was able to tell the ER technicians what to do!"

School-Age Children (age seven to twelve)

If your child is diagnosed with asthma at this relatively late age, it will be more difficult to make the necessary changes in lifestyle, food, and environment because you and your child will have established certain routines and habits. And since you have lived all these years without a diagnosis of asthma, it may also take time for the shock to wear off and for all the family members to accept the news and the new way of life it brings. You may feel tempted to go back to the level of protectiveness and responsibility you felt when your child was smaller. Your life and your child's life will be easier if you can:

- Be a bit more detailed in your explanation of asthma and the Natural Asthma Control Program—show her the illustration of the respiratory system on page 7 in Chapter 1. Reassure her that she is not alone and that there are many other children with asthma who are taking the same medications, vitamin supplements, and herbs as she is.

- Tell her that she should feel free to ask you questions and express her feelings such as fear or concern or confusion.

- Be persistent and consistent in your efforts to ease into lifestyle and dietary changes.

- Make sure, as she becomes more self-sufficient and spends more time away from you, that she understands what she needs to do to control asthma.

- Encourage your child to continue to become more independent and explore the world.

- Allow her to test her limits, within reason. For example, she may want to compete athletically, but to prevent a flare-up she may need to take conventional or natural medicine before practice or an event.

- Increase her level of responsibility for being aware of possible triggers, taking conventional or natural medications, keeping tabs on how much medicine she is taking, and monitoring her condition. Many parents find using a chart and stickers or stars is a fun way to keep track. Supervise your child closely at first, and then gradually let her take over while you just check the chart at the end of the week.

- Prepare your child and her friends for any overnight stays by talking over your child's needs with the host parents and children.

Although some children start to rebel as they get older and become difficult about following the asthma control program, others become remarkably in tune with their bodies and what is and isn't good for them. A good example is James, an eleven-year-old boy who had his first episode when he was fourteen months old and has been on our program for nine years. His mother says he never seemed to mind being on a special diet, and that "now he knows that if he's feeling the twinges of asthma coming on, that too much sugar can put him over the edge." The remarkably mature James says, "The most important advice I could give other kids is to limit everything—even if it's really good. Because there's a point at which it's too much. Everyone I know, including myself, loves sugar, greasy foods—stuff like that. It's good, but you have to limit it. I don't feel deprived, because I'm doing it myself, and because I know the results. I feel bad when I do too much, and better when I don't. I tell my friends, too—some of them listen, some of them don't. Me and the other kids with asthma, we watch out for each other, and let each other know when we're eating too many candy bars."

Adolescence (thirteen years and up)

This is a time of turmoil for your child. At this stage of his life he is intensely testing his limits—and yours—and asserting his independence. Adolescents rebel by refusing to take their medications. Their independence must be respected and encouraged, but not to the point that it is self-destructive. He is thinking about sex and career, and probably wondering how asthma will affect them. By this age, kids are paying attention to their bodies, becoming more confident in their ability to take care of themselves, but paradoxically resentful of being "different." Thus, this time can be a period of relaxation and maturity or frustrating rebelliousness— or both. To help your child make the transition to adulthood with the least amount of emotional turmoil for all, while safeguarding his health, try to:

- Continue to communicate openly with him and encourage him to ask questions about asthma and express his feelings about his condition. Determine whether there are issues that are too difficult for him to discuss with you, and if so, find a physician, teacher, or counselor to whom he can turn.

- Involve him in making decisions about his care, and include him in the discussion during doctor visits— don't treat him as if he weren't there.

- Encourage him to ask questions of you and of his doctor.

- Teach him how to more carefully, precisely, and consistently monitor his symptoms, measure his peak flow levels, and avoid triggers.

- Keep defining the boundaries of responsibility and freedom—when is the ball in his court and when is it in yours?

- When he accepts increasing responsibility for managing asthma, reinforce this by giving him more freedom. By the time he reaches his late teens, your child can be almost completely responsible for his asthma control program.

- Remind him that adhering to the Natural Asthma Control Program gives him more freedom because asthma symptoms are less likely to hold him back. For example, if his room is cluttered and dusty, explain why it is in his best interest to keep it clean and less cluttered. Negotiate about the things he absolutely must have in his room, and let him earn the right to keep them by keeping up with his household chores (such as cleaning the room once a week) or schoolwork.

- Reduce tension around dating by helping him figure ways to avoid potential triggers.

- Talk about the dangers of smoking, drugs, and alcohol for teens with asthma—these can weaken his body and cloud his thinking should he have an episode while under the influence.

ACTION STEP:

CHANGING NEGATIVE FEELINGS

When you're in the middle of an argument or other stressful situation, you feel trapped in your emotions. You can't imagine that you are wrong or that it's possible to react in another way. Yet, there is a way out. It's a technique called cognitive reframing, which forms the basis for many coping strategies. This approach helps you build skills to better manage stress and anxiety. Reframing is basically a matter of changing your attitude so that, with time and practice, you'll evoke a healthier response when you meet a stressful situation.

According to cognitive reframing, people have three choices in the way they respond to stress: positive, negative, or neutral. For example, although no child *likes* to have an asthma episode, some children become very upset and fearful when this happens, while others take it matter-of-factly and remain calm. The same is true of any stressful event—it can be seen as overwhelming or as a challenge that is surmountable.

Through cognitive reframing, you recognize, review, and question your usual way of dealing with something, such as an asthma episode. Then you consciously work on changing the way you perceive and react from negative to positive—or at least to feeling more neutral. The following are common stress reactions to asthma, and some ideas about how you and your child can reframe them.

Assuming the Worst

This is aptly called catastrophizing, and reframing it is called decatastrophizing. Catastrophizing may be an immediate reaction; for example, during a flare-up, you might worry that your child will die. Especially at the beginning, parents wildly overestimate the odds that their child will die. During an asthma flare-up, you or your older children can get caught up in panic mode, spreading fear to your already gasping child. Or you may have a long-term reaction, as when you imagine your child failing at school, being a sickly person, and having a rotten life. It is important to remain calm, confident, and reassuring yourself because children can be sponges for emotions, and your anxiety can be contagious. To reframe this experience, take the following steps.

How to Be Positive During a Flare-up:

- As a parent, learn and teach the whole family what works best during a flare-up. The way you act and the things you say can help break the cycle of fear and anxiety, rather than perpetuate it.

- Be sure to have an action plan that you and your child's doctor have worked out in advance.

- Calm your own body with the breathing and relaxation techniques provided in Chapter 11.

- Calm your mind with positive "self-talk": Repeat to yourself that you and your child are in control of the situation, that you have a plan of action, that you know what to do, that medication is available that will stop the episode, and that you can always call your doctor or go to the emergency room if needed.

- Encourage your child to do breathing exercises along with you.

Teach your child to repeat silently to himself: "I am in control, I know what to do, I can do my breathing exercises, I can take my medicine, I'm not going to die, my mother (or teacher) is here, I'm going to be okay."

How to Be Positive About the Future

- Tell yourself that the odds are highly unlikely your child will die of asthma.

- Tell yourself that you have it under control, and with proper care, including natural therapies, his condition will not worsen—it will improve.

- Realize that once your child's asthma is under better control, asthma will not be an obstacle to his being successful at school and at life.

Feelings About Being "Different"

Your child may be feeling uncomfortably different from his peers—he has to take medicine, perhaps eat differently, constantly be on the lookout for triggers that his friends needn't be concerned about. You may be deeply disappointed that your child isn't perfect, and you may feel guilt that you feel this way. To reframe this experience:

- Encourage your child to talk about any problems he is having at school—are other children teasing him or avoiding him because he has asthma?

- Instead of dwelling on your child's weaknesses, differences, and limitations, look for and emphasize his strengths.

- Reassure your child that he has strengths and capabilities and point out that every child is different and unique.

- Remind your child of all the incredible role models of people with asthma who prove that kids can do a lot of things—even be Olympic champions.

- Encourage your child to re-engage with his friends, to engage in as many activities as in the past, to feel a sense of accomplishment.

- Encourage your child to be part of a group or groups so he feels less isolated and more like he "belongs." For example, consider sending him to a summer camp; depending on your child, he may be able to be mainstreamed to a regular camp, or he may do better in a camp for asthmatic children.

- Encourage your child to join a support group (discussed later in this chapter).

Claudia's mother is a big advocate of honest communication and is grateful that her child's school is helping her child talk about the stresses of feeling different. "At the school she goes to now, they encourage the children to be very verbal, to express their feelings, rather than keep silent," observes her mother. "If there is trouble between two children—if one child is making fun of my child because she gets breathless and has to slow down during playtime—they encourage her to talk to her friend about what hurt her feelings. This seems to be very good for my child." She continues: "Claudia comes home less stressed than she did from her other school. She sleeps better at night. And at home now she tells me if something is bothering her, if there is something she doesn't like, or if I have hurt her feelings in some way. Parents can also do this at home, if they are aware of the importance of reducing stress in their child's life."

Blaming and Anger

Sometimes parents blame themselves or their spouses for their child having asthma, or are angry at their doctors when they are really angry at the condition. Arguments over what your child can and cannot do, and how best to treat her condition, often degenerate into ugly finger-pointing battles. Your child may blame herself for having asthma and feel guilty that she is causing the family trouble and extra expense. To better cope with these emotions:

- Try to put these thoughts and feelings in perspective—the fact that your child has asthma is not your fault, and it does no one any good to scapegoat.

- Reassure your child that you love her, that it's not her fault that she has asthma, and that the whole family will get through this together.

- Acknowledge where your true responsibility lies—in seeing that your child gets the best care, which includes following our Natural Asthma Control Program.

Overprotectiveness

It's natural for you to be concerned and caring and want to help your child when he is in distress. But if you allow this loving instinct to go too far, you run the risk of becoming too doting and overly protective of your child. When your life revolves around your child with asthma, your other children may feel neglected and diminished. Your asthmatic child may feel and behave more sickly. Children naturally crave attention, and get it any way they can, and he's bound to notice that his wheezing, coughing, and struggling to breathe gets him a lot of attention. If you reward him with lots of attention during an episode and grant him special privileges such as staying up later than his siblings, or excusing him from chores, you are reinforcing such "illness behavior." Even if your family is emotionally stable, your child may learn to exaggerate symptoms to get these goodies and to play up his sick role and feel entitled to extra privileges. Ultimately, this way of dealing with things harms everyone. Deep down, kids don't really like to be labeled in this way; they would rather be "normal" and may harbor resentment that can fester and grow. To prevent overprotectiveness and its emotional consequences:

- Watch out that you are not setting unnecessary limits on what your child can do because of your desire to prevent any more flare-ups.

- Think positive. Rather than limiting contact with other children, restricting play, and giving special privileges, come up with creative ways to overcome genuine limitations, minimize them, or substitute another activity. For example, if your child is allergic to animals and wants to play with other children who have pets, suggest that they play outside where there is less dander.

- Treat all your children equally—discipline inappropriate behavior and reward appropriate behavior. Put firm limits in place that are fair to all your children. Although you feel bad for your child who is suffering, it's okay to say no.

- Verbally reward "wellness behavior"—doing breathing exercises, eating well, taking supplements—with praise and attention, not extra privileges.

It's a fine line between reasonable concern and overprotectiveness, a delicate dance that you as a loving parent will be doing for the rest of your life. Lynn, the mother of nine-year-old Anita, who has been on our program for five years now, recalls how she struggled with being overprotective. She says, "When a doctor says to you that your child has asthma, the first feeling you have is to protect her—to make a shield around her. I always have to say to myself, 'Don't go overboard, she needs to be exposed to life.' When we would go to the house of a friend who had cats and a carpet, I would get nervous. My husband, who is more laid back than me would say, 'Hey, relax!' When my daughter started to get better with treatment, I started to relax and be less protective, because I felt secure that this was helping her."

Another parent voices her concern that overprotectiveness could lead to her child being in denial about his condition—the reverse of the little boy who cried wolf. "My son Pierre's father is a musician and one night he had a gig that was about forty minutes away from our home. We all piled into the car, eager to hear him play. A few minutes later, Pierre told us he was having trouble breathing. I turned to his father and said, 'Okay, that's it; we've got to go back and give him a nebulizer treatment. Maybe you should go without us.' My son got upset and pleaded, 'No, no, I want to go.' We realized that the next time something like this comes up he may not tell us he's having trouble because he'll be afraid we'll limit him too much. So, we went home, he had a quick treatment, we drove to the gig together, and we had a great time. I've learned it doesn't pay to be overprotective. Encourage your child to tell you what's going on, and don't overreact—rather, praise him for telling you."

ACTION STEP:

GET INFORMED

Educating yourself, your child, and your family can go a long way in clearing up any misunderstandings and misconceptions that contribute to emotional stress. By giving yourself a foundation of knowledge you help alleviate exaggerated or unfounded feelings of fear, anxiety, and helplessness; open the door to new ways of thinking and reacting which are less stressful; and restore feelings of control and confidence.

Often, it helps to use a variety of media to get and share information. Begin by sharing the information in this book. Buy or borrow some of the videos listed in the "Resources" section; there are now videos geared toward either adults or children that make learning about asthma entertaining. If you have access to the Internet, check out the growing number of Web sites; we have listed a few in the "Resources" section, but to be up-to-date, use a search engine on your own computer or one at your school or library.

Make sure you know as much as you need to about asthma. Your child's doctor can be your greatest source of information and emotional support. Sometimes just sitting down for a half hour with the office nurse can be informative and reassuring and ultimately reduce asthma episodes. There is evidence that education actually saves time in the long run. And research shows that education is a key part of successful asthma treatment. One study, by Noreen Clark of the University of Michigan, demonstrated that communication and education were needed in addition to anti-inflammatory medication to reduce symptoms, hospitalizations, and ER visits.

Educate and Involve Your Child

It's never too early to begin educating your child about asthma, because the sooner he becomes involved in his own care, the better. A well-informed child develops a sense of independence and confidence that he can handle his condition, and this helps ease unfounded fears and anxieties. He is more likely to be aware of the factors that trigger asthma and more likely to avoid them. Earlier in this chapter, we provide you with age-specific guidelines for teaching your child self-care. For example, you can teach even a preschooler to recognize signs of worsening symptoms and to ask for help when needed. We have seen even children as young as three learn to do breathing exercises that can help prevent or alleviate the symptoms of an asthma episode. As your child gets older, you can ask him to remind you when it is time for regularly scheduled medications or natural therapies such as vitamin supplements, and eventually he can do more and more of these on his own.

"You need to make explaining fun, not all serious and stressful like a science project" says Gillian, whose four-year-old was diagnosed with asthma when he was two. "His father and I wanted to encourage him to cough up mucus, so we called it 'chunks of water,' which was something he could understand. This made it less stressful for us, too."

Educate and Involve Your Family

You can teach siblings about asthma, too, and draw them into the asthma control program so they don't feel left out. Show them how they can help, for example, by keeping track of a younger sibling's medications and natural remedies, or by doing the breathing exercises explained in the next chapter. Be sure to thank them for their help and keep them informed of their sibling's condition. This shows that you care about them too, and that you know and appreciate they care.

ACTION STEP:

WORK WITH YOUR CHILD'S SCHOOL

Your child spends most of his day at school, and any problems at home tend to eventually spill into his school life, and vice versa. According to the American Lung Association, asthma is responsible for ten million missed school days every year. Ironically, school conditions themselves can be responsible for some of those missed days. Here are some ways that you can ease any emotional issues surrounding this significant part of your child's emotional, intellectual, and social life.

- Discuss your child's asthma with his teachers, classroom aides, school nurse, counselors, coaches, and principal.

- Provide the school with written instructions on how to spot an emergency and steps to follow should one occur.

- If your child takes medication regularly and needs a dose during school hours, discuss this issue with school personnel and work out a schedule. Many schools require that medications be securely stored, so talk over with your child the fact that he may need to go to the nurse's or principal's office to get his medication. Bear in mind that it is better psychologically and physically if the school allows your child to carry his inhaler with him, assuming he is mature and responsible enough. If adult supervision is required, your child may be embarrassed or be reluctant to take the time and call attention to himself by going to an office. The American College of Allergy and Immunology's official position is that children who are responsible should be allowed to carry their own inhalers.

- Explain to the staff your efforts to reduce symptoms and medication through the use of natural therapies. Discuss ways that school personnel and schoolmates can help your child avoid triggers, follow any special diet, or take any herbs or nutritional supplements that are part of your program.

- Explain firmly that your child needs to avoid certain triggers and provide a list of his triggers. Make sure there is adequate air ventilation. Find out if there is dust, mold, chemical irritants, or allergens such as glue or paint, or animals such as hamsters, gerbils, or parakeets; then work out ways your child can avoid them.

- Since exercise is one of the most common triggers, meet with the physical education instructor or coach and explain that he should be able to participate in any activity, but may need to take medication before or during the activity. If your child is young, tell his teachers to check that your child is wearing a scarf over his mouth during playtime in cold outdoor weather. Gyms are notoriously dusty and pose a problem for any child with asthma and allergies, so request that the floor be mopped each night.

- Work with your child's teacher to discuss ways that your child can make up days missed from school. If your child has a learning problem, find out if it is related to asthma. As your child achieves greater control over his asthma, he will miss fewer and fewer days from school.

- Be prepared to answer any questions your child's classmates may have about asthma. You may want to anticipate their questions by having a talk with them at the beginning of the school year.

- Become a school volunteer; that way, you'll be able to have direct contact with teachers and see exactly what's going on in the school. Having mom or dad around even a few hours a week will also give your child a greater sense of security.

- You needn't do all this alone. For example, Open Airways for Schools, a multimedia program of the American Lung Association, helps teach children, parents, and school personnel about the condition. Another option is the Student Asthma Action Card (SAAC). Designed for use in elementary, middle, and high schools, the SAAC is a tool for parents and physicians to help school personnel understand the individual student's asthma management needs and what to do in case of an emergency. It is available from the Asthma and Allergy Foundation of America (AAFA). (See "Resources" section for addresses and phone numbers.)

When you have a good relationship with your child's school, school can be a tremendous ally. Francesca's mother emphatically believes that "Without the teachers' involvement, you can't do it. They are the ones who can tell you how your child is doing. They are with your child more than you are during the day. Francesca's teachers were very helpful. I explained to them what symptoms to watch out for. They would call me and tell me if she was having even early subtle symptoms such as a rash, a sneeze, or if she was a little cranky. And when I picked her up, I would take a few minutes to talk to them to see if there was anything I should know. That would help me tremendously. This would alert me and give me the opportunity to fine-tune her diet. If she started to show early warning signs, I would, for example, be stricter with her anti-asthma diet and not allow even small amounts of dairy for the next few days. And whenever I had an appointment with Dr. Bock, I had an appointment with the school the next day to tell them about any changes they needed to know about."

Knowing that your child is in good hands while at school can be a tremendous relief, but for some parents it also takes persistence. "When it was time for my son to go off to school, I felt a gut-wrenching fear—what if something happened to him?" says the mother of another of our patients. She continues: "So, I went with him the first day, and when I brought his inhaler to the school nurse, I firmly explained to her that if he says he is having trouble breathing and needs treatment, she needs to pay attention. He is not fooling around. And if he needs treatment, I must be notified." She adds, "You need to take it upon yourself to inform

CHILD CARE

Having someone else take care of your child brings up many issues and stresses. It's hard enough to find qualified care when you have a healthy child, and when you add asthma to the picture it gets more complicated. New people, new places, and other children expose your child to potential triggers. Caregivers may not understand asthma or why you are adamant they take certain measures. When choosing child care—be that a day care center, sitter, or nanny, these tips will help ease your mind and protect your child's well-being:

- Encourage the caregiver to ask questions.
- Make sure he or she is ready to take on the extra responsibility of caring for a child with asthma.
- Specify that you need a nonsmoker who comes to your home or a facility that does not have smokers or pets (if your child is allergic) and is clean enough to avoid allergens such as dust mites and mold.
- Be sure the caregiver understands asthma and knows your child's triggers (for example, perfumes can be a trigger in some children), medication needs, and signs of asthma.
- Remind him or her that other children may not share their food if your child is allergic to it.
- Give the caregiver written instructions for what to do in case of an emergency and written permission to seek and sign for medical help if your child has a flare-up.

Provide the caregiver with an alarm clock to remind him or her when it's time to give your child regularly scheduled medication or natural therapy.

everyone—you can't just rely on the school nurse. I personally talked to his teacher, the principal, the librarian, his art teacher, his music teacher—everyone he came into contact with." At first, her efforts were only partially successful. The first time he needed treatment, he got it. But she was not notified—her son told her himself. "So the next day I read them the riot act. I made it quite clear that I was to be informed. I've never had a problem since, and my stress level has gone way down."

Of course, it helps to reward good teacher behavior, just as it helps to reward good behavior in your child. As Francesca's mother notes, "I think it's important to give them reinforcement and to show that I appreciate their vigilance, so I keep telling them 'I love you'—and I mean it!"

ACTION STEP:

GETTING SUPPORT

When should you consider going outside your home for support and counseling? You should consider outside help if your child is suffering from depression or anxiety (see box, "Does Your Child Need Help?", page 206) or despite your efforts you are unable to cope and communicate with your family members, which blocks change and progress.

Today there are psychotherapists who specialize in chronic illnesses such as asthma, and there are support groups for children with asthma, their parents, and their siblings.

Support and Therapy Groups

As a parent of a child with asthma, you need to take care of yourself, for your sake and for your child's sake. You may feel isolated and in need of practical advice about avoiding triggers, monitoring symptoms, and integrating natural therapies into the asthma control program. The last thing you need is to feel all alone and frustrated in your efforts. A support group of other parents of asthmatic children provides something no doctor or friend can—they are people who have been there and who understand what you are going through. Usually a mixture of seasoned veterans and rookie parents, a group can guide you through the journey—empathize with your fear and anxieties, give you practical information and share experiences and feelings so you feel less alone and advice so you feel less helpless. There are also concrete physical benefits: a 1993 Kaiser-Permanente study found support groups can cut the number of asthma-related doctor visits in half; in a similar 1992 study at San Francisco State University, 80 percent of participants reduced frequency of attacks, doctor visits, and medications.

If there isn't a support group in your area, consider forming one yourself. These groups often grow from seeds sown when parents begin talking in the doctor's waiting room. Support groups for asthmatic children and their families exist in many communities—check with your doctor, the local Lung Association chapter, Mothers of Asthmatic Children, and medical centers. Also check electronic sources for online "chat rooms" and groups.

Counseling

Professional counseling can help clear roadblocks to change. Individual therapy for your child helps him more freely express any concerns he has about asthma. Couples or family counseling can help family members communicate and provides an objective sounding board for issues too painful and complicated to solve outside the professional arena. It helps to realize that big changes—divorce, death of a person close to the child, or moving to another city—can be extra stressful and that therapy may be useful during such times of loss and transition. For example,

DOES YOUR CHILD NEED HELP?

Seek professional help if your child shows any of the following signs of anxiety or depression:

Major signs of anxiety:

- unwilling to be separated from parents, clingy, dependent
- fearfulness, phobias
- physical signs of anxiety such as bedwetting, nail biting
- frequently tells you that he is afraid or nervous
- sleep disturbances—nightmares, inability to fall asleep
- hypochondria or hypervigilance—excessive concern about every little ache and pain

Major signs of depression:

- withdrawal and difficulty socializing with friends
- irritability
- anger
- sadness that doesn't go away
- overeating or undereating
- inability to enjoy the things he used to
- sleep disturbances—too much, too little, waking up in the middle of the night
- difficulty at school; for example, sudden drops in grades, preoccupation with other thoughts, lethargy

during a separation or divorce your child may think that she is such a burden to you and your spouse that she may have caused this terrible rift. Or her brothers and sisters may blame her for the troubles. As a parent, you may subconsciously blame the asthma, too, particularly when it has been the trigger of disagreement and strife. Any major stress in the family will pull your attention away from your child, and she may suffer in the process. During these times, you may find counseling to be particularly useful for yourself, your family, and your child who may otherwise suffer worse asthma symptoms from the stress.

In closing, asthma is a family affair, but it does not have to be all stress and anguish. When you deal with this challenge successfully, it can actually strengthen the bonds between family members and bring you closer to your child. As one mother told us, "You get into an unusually close relationship with a child with asthma. You notice every little thing, because it helps you take good care of him. For instance, I noticed that my child's feet would get cold during an episode, because they were getting less oxygen. Sometimes I would put him in a warm bath because the steam would relieve his coughing and the water would warm his feet. Or I would tell him to crawl into bed with me, which would warm him all over and the close body contact would relax him and slow and calm his breathing. When he was in the hospital, and he had an intravenous needle in him, I had him sleeping on top of me. I was in very close, intense contact for long periods of time, and although I wish he didn't have asthma, I wouldn't trade those intimate moments for anything."

Next, we show you how the body affects the mind, and vice-versa, and how you and your child can use breathing and other techniques to deal with the stresses of asthma and everyday living by taking advantage of the mind-body connection.

TEN   <u>MIND-BODY MEDICINE</u>

In the previous chapter, we showed how emotions affect asthma, and vice versa, and provided ways to manage toxic emotions through psychology. Another way to influence the mind-body connection is by working with the body. In our experience, we have time and again seen how easy it is for children (and their parents) to learn to physically relax and thus calm feelings of fear and anxiety.

This chapter teaches you some basic relaxation techniques that are useful for your child and for anyone in the family who is feeling stressed. We first describe techniques that you can learn and perform on your own, including breathing techniques, muscle relaxation, massage, and guided imagery. We also provide suggestions for using herbs and homeopathic remedies to help you or your child deal with stress. We then describe several useful techniques that require professional expertise and supervision. If your child uses these techniques regularly, they act as a preventive to stabilize the immune system, reduce the number of episodes and improve quality of life. Used as treatment when symptoms flare, they can calm the fear and decrease the panic that sometimes spirals out of control, thereby reducing the intensity and length of the flare-up.

One of the nicest things about the mind-body therapies is that you can do them together with your children. When you breathe deeply and rhythmically along with your child, both of you become calmer and share the experience of becoming less fearful and more relaxed. When you give your child a massage, you create a special kind of closeness that only loving physical contact can bring. And these techniques can be fun—as, for example, when you play breathing games, or when you bend yourselves into the pretzel positions of yoga. As one mother joyfully told us, "My daughter Francesca takes yoga and loves it. She usually can't wait to get home to show me, to teach me. When the Saturday classes start, I'm going to take yoga with her."

> **REMINDER:** When you take any of the steps in this chapter, remember to continue your child's regular medical treatment. Do not reduce asthma medications on your own—do this only under the advice and supervision of your child's physician. If your child shows any of the danger signs of an asthma flare-up (see page 59, Chapter 4), seek medical attention immediately.

RELAXING THE BODY, CALMING THE MIND

The nervous system is involved in the stress response as well as the relaxation response. The nervous system controls breathing in several ways. It controls the diameter of the bronchi, through contracting and relaxing the bronchial muscles encircling them. The part of the nervous system responsible is the *autonomic (involuntary) nervous system*. There are two parts of the autonomic nervous system: the *sympathetic nervous system* (which tenses you up for action) and the *parasympathetic nervous system* (which slows down functions and helps the body heal).

The rate of breathing is also controlled by nerves in the chest cavity that end at the rib muscles and diaphragm. The nerves are sensitive to the amount of carbon dioxide in the blood. The higher the concentration of carbon dioxide, the more the nerves become stimulated, and the faster the breathing rate. As we have seen in the previous chapter, mental stress can affect the body and worsen asthma by constricting the airways and compromising the immune system.

Stress causes your body to be on the alert, but mind-body techniques break the cycle of fear—they relax the muscles and signal your body to step down production of stress hormones. During relaxation, the sympathetic nervous system withdraws and the parasympathetic nervous system takes its place. Your body gets a signal that it's safe to calm down. Once your muscles relax, the rest of you realizes that it can relax too. This in turn relaxes the airways and allows the immune system to function more normally.

ACTION STEP:

BREATHING EXERCISES

Breathing is what asthma is all about, and breathing exercises are the cornerstone of many of the the mind-body therapies in this chapter. Most people are in the habit of taking shallow breaths of air that fill only the top part of their lungs. In individuals with asthma this tendency is exaggerated. This breathing pattern is not desirable because eventually it disrupts the normal functions of the body and reinforces feelings of anxiety. It limits your child's intake of oxygen and encourages her body to develop either a caved-in chest appearance or a barrel chest.

On the other hand, taking deep breaths that more fully inflate and deflate the lungs allows a thorough exchange of stale air for fresh, oxygenated air. It conditions your child's chest muscles, lungs, and airways and allows her to develop a healthier posture. It helps her engage in physical activity. And it can be supremely relaxing, giving her immune system a break. In fact, a University of Massachusetts Medical Center study showed that a similar breathing practice to that provided here reduces asthma attacks.

In our health centers we often rely on biofeedback (discussed later in the chapter) as a tool to help children learn proper breathing and relaxation, but many of our patients are able to learn them without such high-tech devices. We have found that the techniques are more effective if parents learn them first and then teach them to their children, and if both participate in the activity. Be sure to first teach and practice the exercises when your child is relaxed and symptom free. And be sure you are relaxed and low-key about it, too! Jimmy's mother says, "We don't call it yoga breathing or abdominal breathing—we call it simply 'good breathing.' I just tell my son to breathe deeply, and try to slow it down if he can. We use it if he notices early warning signs of an impending flare-up—if he's been playing hard—or if he is taking medicine through a nebulizer. I think this is one way he can tell his body that it's okay, that he can relax."

The following breathing techniques are progressive, with each technique building on the previous one. They are based on diaphragmatic breathing, which you may be familiar with if you practice yoga. This involves lowering the diaphragm, the muscle that separates the lungs from the abdominal cavity, which allows the entire chest to expand. Breathe through your nose (unless it is stuffed up) for the entire time you do the exercise.

1. Long, Slow Breathing

This simple preliminary technique helps introduce the concept and the feeling of breathing more slowly than most people are used to. Simply lie down in a calm quiet place and breathe normally through your nose. Inhale slowly through your nose for a count of five or more. Then exhale slowly for a count of five. Repeat several times, continuing to breathe through your nose, not your mouth, and notice how relaxing this is. Practice this two or three times a day until it becomes second nature.

2. Deep Breathing

The next phase is to combine the long, slow inhale and exhale with correct use of the diaphragm. Again lying down, place one hand over your chest and the other on your abdomen. Exhale as much air as is comfortable, contracting your diaphragm and allowing your abdomen to sink down and push the air out of your lower lungs and then the middle and top of the lungs. If you are doing this correctly, you will see that the hand on your abdomen lowers quite a bit and the hand on your chest moves very little.

Next, inhale deeply and slowly, allowing your abdomen to puff up so you fill the lower lungs. Again watch to see that the hand on your abdomen rises, indicating that you are breathing diaphragmatically. This may take several tries for some people—in children and adults it may help to imagine your torso is a balloon.

Exhale slowly, first emptying your chest and then your abdominal area. Repeat the inhalation and exhalation, trying to slow the breath even more. This should feel like a wave of air rhythmically entering and leaving your body. Only breathing in should require any effort—allow the air to flow out on its own as you let the weight of your abdomen relax down.

The goal is to extend the exhale for as long as you can, while keeping the inhale to a count of two. In our health center, we usually aim for six cycles a minute. A cycle is one inhale and one exhale. (The "normal" rate of breathing is about twenty cycles per minute.) Kids usually enjoy counting and seeing the progress they are making. One variation that children seem to like is to place an object on their tummies—a small book perhaps—so they can have fun making it go up and down. You and your child can turn this into a game, trying to see who can exhale the longest. Eventually, do this exercise sitting up, and then standing. Practice for a total of ten minutes a day and see what a difference it makes in the way you and your child feel—in the freedom and expansiveness you feel in your chest and your breath.

3. The Walking Breath

The final phase is to do diaphragmatic breathing while walking. Take your child for an easy ten- or fifteen-minute walk, concentrating on taking deep, slow breaths. Again, try to extend the exhale but keep the inhale to a count of two. This will help your child get accustomed to doing this type of breathing during normal everyday activities, and eventually, during more strenuous exercise.

MAKE BREATHING FUN

Young children are more likely to go along with learning this type of breathing if you can turn it into a game. We hope you will use your own imagination and let your surroundings give you ideas, but you might start out with simply having your child blow common everyday objects. Have her blow a Ping-Pong ball or a pencil across a tabletop. A candle flame is another satisfying target; move it farther and farther away as her lungs get stronger. Blow up balloons together, blow soap bubbles, and encourage her to learn to play a musical wind instrument such as a harmonica, flute, or saxophone. Singing is another pleasurable way for your child to exercise her lungs and learn diaphragmatic control.

Remember, too, that swimming is an excellent exercise for an asthmatic child, in part because it encourages rhythmic forceful breathing. Just floating is a good practice as well, because this teaches your child how to relax, and she will be able to translate this sensation to dry land when needed.

ACTION STEP:

PROGRESSIVE MUSCLE RELAXATION

This technique builds on the series of breathing exercises learned in the previous action step. It involves tensing and then relaxing the muscles of the body, which creates a state of deep relaxation. It effectively slows the breathing and heart rate, instilling a state of deep relaxation. Give yourself a half hour to begin, and as you become adept, you may reduce the time to twenty or fifteen minutes. Begin in a warm, quiet room free of distractions.

1: Lying down, close your eyes and take a few deep breaths. Begin the deep breathing exercise described above (#2) and try to maintain it throughout the relaxation.

2: Focus your attention on your feet and point your toes very hard. Hold for ten seconds and then let them go completely limp for twenty seconds. Work up your legs by flexing and relaxing your feet, tensing and relaxing your calves, and then tensing your thighs by pulling up your kneecaps and then letting them go, enjoying the contrast between the two sensations.

3: Now squeeze and relax your buttocks, waist, back, chest, right hand and arm, left hand and arm, shoulders, neck, and scalp. Include your face, opening your mouth and eyes wide, then scrunching them tight before completely relaxing those muscles.

4: Finally, stretch your arms and legs to their longest length, and elongate every muscle in between. Let go one more time.

5: Return your attention to your breathing and your surroundings, opening your eyes.

Once you are comfortable with the technique, aim to tense the muscle for ten seconds and let it relax for twenty seconds. With each muscle relaxation, say the word *relax* to yourself and imagine the tension melting away like butter or like steam escaping from a vent. Be conscious of how different the relaxation feels from the tension. Eventually, you will no longer need to tense the muscle before you relax it; just think of each body part and think the word *relax*.

ACTION STEP:

GUIDED IMAGERY

Guided imagery is used in conjunction with the above relaxation techniques and is a way of translating positive thoughts into mental images in order to achieve a specific result. Long used by competitive athletes to visualize their victory and give them a winning edge, this technique is now being used by medical patients to visualize health and wellness.

Because it involves using the imagination to create internal visual images and requires suggestibility, children are particularly adept. They can use it to improve immunity, resist infection, and open up bronchioles. Recent research by Georgetown University psychologist Mary Banks Gregerson had subjects imagine their white blood cells attacking and ingesting weakened cold and flu viruses. When they focused on their blood, sure enough—blood lymphocytes went up. When they focused on their saliva, an immune component particular to saliva rose. In a recent study, children aged six to twelve were taught to do guided visualization; they were able to successfully raise their IgA levels, a component of the immune system. In addition, this technique has allowed asthmatics to reduce medication and go months without an attack.

You can lead your child in guided imagery to help her marshal her immune system's forces or to relax her airways. She first needs to put herself in a state of deep relaxation using one of the techniques described above. Then, help her create her own unique image of what she wants to happen, helping her "see" every little detail to make it more real. Parents usually do this instinctively— it's like telling a story. For example, in our practice we often use this imagery, which is good for opening up bronchioles:

"Imagine you are going down a staircase to a beautiful sunny beach, lots of your friends are there, your mom, your dad, everyone is having a really nice day. Feel the warmth of the sun, smell the salty water, the sand beneath your feet. Your breathing is slow, smooth, and easy, your lungs are like big balloons with lots of space for air, they are filling and emptying, filling and emptying, filling and emptying."

Guide her through this imagery once a day. We find that the best time for everyone is at night, just before bedtime.

ACTION STEP:

BREATHING FOR SYMPTOM RELIEF

Often, what happens during an asthma flare-up is the opposite of the long, slow diaphragmatic breathing you've just learned. When your child has trouble getting enough air, panic can set in and your child instinctively breathes quickly and shallowly, using the upper lungs only. But this actually makes symptoms worse, breathing becomes even more difficult, creating more anxiety and more rapid, shallow breathing in a never-ending cycle that requires medication to break. Using slow, rhythmic breathing during the beginning of an episode may eliminate the panic and ultimately accomplish the same thing as medication.

Most children can eventually learn to do slow, rhythmic

breathing on their own during an episode, but, particularly with a younger child, it helps if you work on this technique together. When your child is starting to have a flare-up, take her into a quiet room, if possible. Lie or sit down together, and match her breathing pattern, which at first will be rapid and shallow. Then, gradually, begin to slow down and deepen your own exhale and inhale, and tell your child to try to breathe the way you are. It may help to put your hand on her abdomen to check that she is breathing diaphragmatically. Slowly and progressively extend the exhale as you did during the practice sessions, until your child is relaxed and has reached the normal breathing rate of about twenty breaths per minute. (During an episode it may reach as high as eighty breaths.)

Depending on the severity of the flare-up, it may take up to twenty minutes to restore normal breathing. You may eventually add some form of guided imagery, described above, or massage, described below, to this practice. Other forms of natural therapy such as herbs and homeopathy are complementary to this technique and may have a synergistic effect. Remember, if your child continues to panic and have trouble breathing despite these efforts, don't hesitate to administer asthma medication.

ACTION STEP:

MASSAGE

Being touched and held with affection is one of life's simplest and most basic needs. It is also one of the oldest natural therapies. Massage, which is a structured, skilled way of touching, has become a legitimate area of scientific study, and today there's even an entire institute devoted to the study and promotion of touch—the Touch Research Institute at the University of Miami. The institute is helping to document that massage not only feels good—it does good. Recent research supports the use of many forms of touching, from Swedish massage to Chinese acupressure to therapeutic touch, to help relieve symptoms of pain and stress, enhance immunity, and alleviate anxiety and mild to moderate depression. Scientists have confirmed by measurement that massage reduces muscle tension; they have also documented that massage increases IgA—the immune system protein your body uses to fight a cold.

In a landmark study of premature infants, those who received a firm fifteen-minute massage three times a day gained 47 percent more weight than babies who were merely touched or cuddled. The massaged infants also went home an average of six days sooner. In India, infants are massaged every day from the day they are born to age three, and weekly after that. By age six, children are massaging their elders. It's common for entire families to massage each other once a week. Pregnant women are massaged daily during pregnancy and for over a month after giving birth.

As far as we know, there are no studies on massage and asthma in children, but in our clinical experience we have seen how beneficial it can be. Fortunately, you don't need to be a pro to give a caring, healing, relaxing massage. There are several studies using nonprofessionals, including parents massaging their children, which show that basic strokes using steady pressure are all that's needed. Massage can profoundly affect your child's state of health by relieving stress and perhaps boosting immunity. Massage is also very relaxing for the parent who is giving it and helps form stronger bonds, helping children feel more loved and secure. There are many good massage books and videotapes available to get you started, such as *Massage for Healthier Children* by Marybetts Sinclair (Wingbow Press, 1992). To make sure your child gets the most from a massage, encourage her to breathe deeply and slowly, inhaling and exhaling in sync with the massage strokes, and to tell you what feels good and what feels uncomfortable. If she becomes restless, stop. Either start again when she has settled down or give her a big hug and save the massage for another time.

If massage is not for you or your child, remember, just holding, cuddling, kissing, and gently rocking your child, and the feelings of love and security this brings, will be comforting enough to relax your child, relieve anxiety, and enhance her immune system.

Massage for Symptom Relief

You may also help reduce the severity of an asthma flare-up by using the following specialized techniques. They work to relax the chest and back muscles to help the air flow more easily. Unlike preventive massage, they are performed with your child sitting up because it is usually easier for her to breath when upright. Practice on your child when she is symptomless or on adults or other children beforehand so you are ready when a flare-up occurs. You can repeat these as often as necessary during an episode.

1. Scapular Massage

Have your child sitting with her back toward you (on your knee, if she is small). With one hand, hold her firmly under the arm. With the thumb of your free hand, make fifty to one hundred firm, gentle strokes along one shoulder blade, in the space between the inner edge of the shoulder blade and the spinal column. Repeat with the other side. This should take about five minutes.

2. Chest Massage

With your child sitting facing you (sitting on your knee, if she is small), hold her firmly under the arm with one hand. With the thumb of the other hand, stroke gently from the middle of her chest toward her nipple. Then switch sides. This should take a total of about five minutes.

3. Shoulder Point

Depending on her height, have your child stand or sit with her back to you. Place your index finger on the point midway between his neck and shoulder. Press firmly, making small circular motions. Your child may be somewhat uncomfortable during this vigorous treatment, but if you keep at it, you may ease symptoms.

ACTION STEP:

YOGA

Yoga means union of mind and body and consists of physical and mental exercises, or "poses." Yoga includes breathing techniques based on diaphragmatic breathing and helps relax the mind and body, restore balance to the immune system, and strengthen and open the chest and lungs. Many studies with adults and one with children with asthma showed significant improvement—less medication, fewer bronchial spasms, less anxiety about the condition, and fewer exercise-induced attacks—with regular yoga practice. There are several books and tapes that feature yoga techniques that have been adapted to children's interests, needs, and abilities, For example, the videotape *YogaKids* by Living Arts (800-2-LIVING). They also make tapes for adults.

HERBS AND HOMEOPATHY TO REDUCE STRESS

Using medicines to reduce stress and anxiety has a long history. Today, conventional medicine, for example, treats stress with antianxiety and tranquilizing drugs such as Valium. However, these may be habit forming and impose unwanted side effects. Instead, you may want to treat stress—both the initial psychological stress as well as the way your body responds physiologically—with herbs or homeopathy, which are gentler on the system, yet just as effective.

Herbal Stress Relief Formula.

There are a number of stress-relief formulas available that may help. Or you can make your own formula using the following herbs:

- Valerian
- Damiana
- Hops

Use equal parts of all three herbs and follow the instructions for mixing and using herbal formulas given on page 156 in Chapter 8. If this formula make you or your child too drowsy (a boon if you use before bedtime, but not if you use during the day), substitute two parts vervain for the hops.

Homeopathic Stress Remedies.

There are also combination homeopathic remedies useful for relieving stress. You may want to try Boereke & Tafel's *Alfalco*, a tonic for relief of fatigue and insomnia from nervousness, overwork, stress, and tension or *Sedalia*, a similar preparation from Boiron. Take as directed on the label. Or try one of the following single remedies, following the guidelines on pages 169–170 in Chapter 8:

- *Pulsatilla*—for touchy, sensitive individuals who react by being anxious, sad, weepy, and dependent. Especially useful during adolescence and menopause in women who are moody, struggling with mood swings, whiny and clingy, and don't tolerate heat well.

- *Kali phosphoricum*—this is a general nerve tonic that is a powerful "soother." Best for those times when you feel you've been through an emotional wringer, you are mentally and physically exhausted, everything is just too difficult, and you've just "had it."

- *Sepia*—for tense, weepy, irritable types who are depressed, and "down," feel utterly worn out, and look pale and wan, with dark circles under the eyes. Your body feels heavy, and you feel better temporarily after eating or vigorous exercise.

ACTION STEP:

WORKING WITH A PROFESSIONAL

Some relaxation techniques, such as biofeedback and hypnosis, require or are best done with the help of a professional. We offer both at our health centers, but you may need to ask your child's physician for a referral to a reputable practitioner.

Biofeedback

This technique involves using a device that monitors and measures physical responses so your child has concrete evidence that she is breathing deeply and slowly. It gives feedback in the form of sounds or lights so that learning to breath correctly is more like acquiring a physical skill such as hitting a tennis ball, where you see and hear the results through trial and error and practice. Usually a person uses this technique to learn to relax, but it has also been used to reverse allergic responses and to relieve asthma. For example, a 1992 study of biofeedback in asthma patients at San Francisco State University demonstrated that 80 percent of participants reported fewer episodes and visits to the emergency room, and less use of medication. Eventually, the person learns to elicit these responses without using the device.

Hypnosis

Hypnosis is a trance state that, in a sense, is similar to daydreaming. Some people also compare it to becoming absorbed by music to the extent that you are unaware of anything else. Hypnosis is useful in children with asthma because it enhances their ability to relax and absorb positive suggestions. For example, a suggestion we might use is, "As you relax, your breathing will become easier and easier." Once your child has been hypnotized and given the appropriate suggestions, she can be taught to hypnotize herself to relax and reinforce the suggestions given by the hypnotist.

In several studies, hypnotherapy and self-hypnosis have been shown to improve immunity and reduce the frequency and severity of asthma flare-ups. In one study, one group of people were taught relaxation and another received hypnotherapy, 42 percent of the relaxation group improved and 50 percent of the hypnosis group improved. In another similar study, relaxation helped 43 percent and hypnosis helped 59 percent.

ACTION STEP:

ACUPRESSURE FOR SYMPTOM RELIEF

Chinese medicine may be the ultimate mind-body therapy, since the Chinese have always considered the mind and the body to be one. Acupressure, along with acupuncture and herbal therapy, is part of the practice of Chinese medicine. About 25 percent of our practice involves Chinese medicine. We have found it to be extremely effective for treating conditions of imbalance, when nothing structurally is wrong with a child, as is the case with asthma. We find that children are willing to take herbs, but don't like needles. Acupuncture and herbal therapy are generally best left to professionals, but acupuncture's needle-free counterpart, acupressure, is a technique suitable for home care.

Acupressure is the painless, self-care version of acupuncture—you use your fingertip to press the point, rather than a needle. To perform acupressure on your child, see that she is in a relaxed state by doing some deep breathing beforehand. Begin by briefly placing your palm over the area. Then use the tip of your index or middle finger or thumb to apply the basic technique of pressure and rotation. As you begin pressing, bore into the point rotating your finger in a tight circle. You know you're on the point if your child says the point feels tender, tingly, or slightly uncomfortable. Press firmly for about one minute, then ease up for a few seconds and apply pressure again. You can work each point for five or ten minutes. Soothe your child with calming words and tell her to exhale slowly as you release the pressure. The following points, also shown in the accompanying illustration, may be useful in preventing or treating asthma.

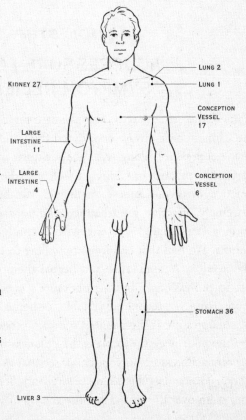

Acupressure points for stimulating the immune system and relieving lung congestion:

Large Intestine 4: On middle of fleshy mound between thumb and forefinger.
Large Intestine 11: At outer end of fold of elbow.
Kidney 27: In hollow below collarbone, where it meets breastbone.
Lung 1: In hollow below collarbone, where it meets shoulder.
Lung 2: One-half-inch above Lung 1.
Conception Vessel 17: On breastbone, in line with nipples.
Conception Vessel 6: One inch below navel.
Stomach 36: Four fingers below lower end of kneecap, on outer surface of leg bone.
Liver 3: In web beween first and second toes, about one inch in.

To Relieve Stuffy Nose, Colds, Flu

A cold, flu, or allergy can cause a stuffy nose, which in turn leads to mouth breathing and bronchospasms. These points help clear your child's nose and sinuses so she can nose breathe, and thus heat and humidify the air before it reaches the lungs. Press Bladder 2, Stomach 6, Large Intestine 20. If her whole head feels congested, try also Large Intestine 4.

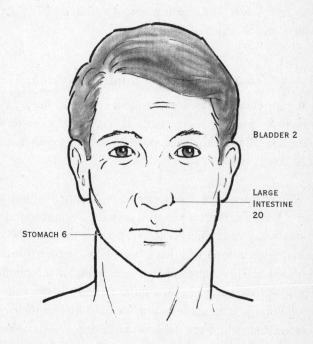

Pressing these acupressure points can help relieve stuffy nose, colds, and flu:

Bladder 2: On ridge of eye socket, one-third out from inner point of eyebrow.
Large Intestine 20: In crease of nostril.
Stomach 6: At angle of jaw.

To Relieve Lung Congestion

These help relieve the congestion associated with asthma symptoms. Press Lung 1, Lung 2, and Conception Vessel 17. These points will ease chest tension, allowing your child to cough deeply and loosen the mucus.

To Relieve Allergies

To relieve allergies which can often trigger asthma, press Large Intestine 4, Liver 3, Large Intestine 11, Kidney 27, Conception Vessel 6, and Stomach 36.

To Stimulate the Immune System

If your child suffers from frequent colds and flu, try preventing them by pressing these points at least once a day during the cold season: Kidney 27, Conception Vessel 17, Conception Vessel 6, and Stomach 36.

This chapter ends the presentation of our Natural Asthma Control Program. But for you, it is only the beginning. In the next and final chapter of this book, you'll meet the parents of three children with asthma who have been following our program for several years. They represent just a sampling of the hundreds of parents we have guided in their quest to find a better solution for their children's asthma. Together, we have helped their children get better and reduce the need for harsh drugs. Today, these children and their parents are living more normal, less stressful lives. They have come far, but remember: They were once in your position and they, too, had to begin somewhere.

ELEVEN

REAL-LIFE SUCCESS STORIES

Knowing about avoiding triggers, improving your child's diet, the benefits of nutritional supplements, herbs, homeopathy, and the importance of emotional support is one thing. Putting it all into practice is another. You may feel as though you are sailing into uncharted territory, but in fact, many parents have made the journey before you. In this chapter, the parents of three of our patients tell you their stories. Through the use of natural therapies, they were able to help their children gradually rebuild their health. As they persisted and grew more knowledgeable and confident, they were able to reduce their child's use of conventional drugs and break the vicious cycle of infection, antibiotics, toxic overload, and asthma.

It is our hope that in reading their stories, you will feel less alone in your desire to give your child something more than conventional medicine alone can provide. You'll see how parents like you learned how to tailor and follow our natural asthma control program, and how children became more and more knowledgeable and responsible for their own care. And you'll find proof that integrating natural therapies with conventional medicine not only works—it works superbly.

ALEX

Alex's mother brought her to us when she was only two years old. By that tender age she had already had several courses of antibiotics for ear infections and was taking two asthma medications. It was clear to us that her immune system was overwhelmed by the multiple infections and conventional drugs her doctor prescribed. Tests showed she had several food allergies worsened by a systemic yeast infection, so our primary strategy was to put her on an antiyeast medication and have her follow a strict antiyeast, hypoallergenic diet. We also prescribed nutritional supplements to fortify her system and help her detoxify, and echinacea to boost her resistance to infection. Since Alex had a lot of mucus in her chest, we added an expectorant syrup to the plan. Alex also had environmental allergies, so her parents made changes in her home environment to minimize exposure to allergens such as dust mites. Fortunately, Alex cooperated fully with this plan and today she can maintain control over her asthma with a less strict program.

Her mother, Marie, says, "Alex was a vibrant, healthy child until I stopped nursing her at the age of six months. That's when the ear infections started. She was getting one almost every month, always after a cold. I was frantic, constantly making office visits, always on the phone. Why was my baby always so sick? My pediatrician's only answer was that this was normal for the cold climate in which we lived. But I didn't like his fatalistic attitude; I felt dissatisfied with his care and began to search for someone else.

"When Alex was sixteen months old, my husband and I made a trip to our home country of France and took her with us. There, we found a homeopathic doctor who told us to give her only goat's milk because it forms less mucus than milk from a cow. He also treated her with a homeopathic remedy. This strategy seemed to help—she didn't get any ear infections the whole time we were there.

"Then, back in the U.S., at eighteen months she took a turn for the worse. At first, we thought that she had a bad bronchitis: she had a lot of trouble breathing, her eyes were all puffy, and her face was very pale. We rushed to an emergency pediatrician who advised us to take her to the hospital. Alex ended up being diagnosed with asthma and spending three days at the hospital. They gave her antibiotics for the bronchitis and started her on albuterol for the asthma. They also put her in an oxygen tent to help her breathe. I was so frightened, I crawled into the tent with her so that our nearness could comfort both of us.

ALEX'S ASTHMA CONTROL PROGRAM

- environmental controls (no wall-to-wall carpeting, non-toxic household cleaners, HEPA air filter)
- hypoallergenic, antiyeast diet
- antiyeast medication
- high-fiber supplement powder
- multi-vitamin-mineral supplement
- vitamin C supplement
- calcium supplement
- echinacea
- herbal expectorant syrup
- homeopathic remedy for allergies
- combination herbal remedy for colds and flu

"From then on, every time she caught a cold she would develop asthma within two days of the first cold symptoms. Fortunately, my search for a progressive physician paid off: when she was twenty-three months old, I found Dr. Bock through a colleague of my husband's. Alex has improved so much under his care that I have stopped seeing the conventional pediatrician except for well-baby checkups."

Detoxifying and Building Strength

At the Rhinebeck Center, we tested Alex for food allergies and found out she was allergic to many common foods: oranges; peanuts; yeast; chocolate; and goat, cow, and soy milk. We also found that she had an overgrowth of yeast in her intestinal tract (candidiasis) because her body had been abused by one course of antibiotics after another. This meant she needed a diet that was low in sugar and refined carbohydrates, including white flour.

We felt the best way for Alex to begin to strengthen her health was to put her on a strict hypoallergenic, antiyeast diet. We told her parents that if they could keep Alex free of ear infections by sticking to this diet for at least one full year, it would mean that her immune system had been built up and her intestinal flora was more balanced. We assured them that she would eventually be able to go on a less restricted diet. But for now—they would need to be very strict. They agreed to give it a try.

Right away, Marie discovered just how difficult it is to avoid certain foods, especially peanuts and yeast, which are ingredients in many prepared foods. We also wanted Alex to avoid grape juice, another common ingredient, because of its high sugar content. Marie recalls, "After Dr. Bock gave me the results of the food allergen test, I spent about four hours in the supermarket, looking at the ingredient labels. It took me that long to find the things that she could have. No canned foods, nothing with food coloring . . . there wasn't much she could eat. So I started cooking everything she ate at home from scratch."

The way Marie dealt with her child's food allergies is a testament to a parent's love and ingenuity. Alex was going to day care at fourteen months, while both parents were in graduate school. Since Marie discovered that this is an age when children want to eat only what their friends are eating, this could have been a problem. But Marie asked the school to provide her with the menus in advance. She then made the same things at home with nonaller-genic ingredients and gave them to the teachers each morning to give Alex later that day. "For example, pizza is a common thing for kids to eat, but Alex couldn't have it because the dough contained refined wheat flour and yeast," she says. "So I used to buy potato flour and make the dough at home. She was allergic to most cheeses, but since I took the other things out of her diet, she could handle small amounts of mozzarella or Swiss cheese, which I sprinkled on top of her pizza."

Food was just the beginning of Alex's Natural Asthma Control Program. Since she also had yeast overgrowth, we pre-scribed Nystatin, an antiyeast medication, which she took for a short time, and a high-fiber powder to help restore her intestinal health. She took a multivitamin supplement, plus extra vitamin C, as well as calcium because she was not drinking milk.

"I used only natural remedies for all her little ailments," notes her mother. "I used an herbal formula that includes echinacea to boost her immunity—she took this every day in the morning. She also began taking a natural expectorant three times a day. During the allergy season, I gave her a homeopathic remedy, or if she had a cold I gave her a natural herbal pill for that as well. These seemed to keep the allergy or cold from getting worse and trigger-ing an asthma attack."

Changes at Home

The family made some changes at home to reduce environ-mental allergens as well. Instead of wall-to-wall carpeting, they have area rugs scattered about the house, except in Alex's room. To keep Alex's otherwise bare wood floor comfortable during the cold winters, her parents came up with this innovative solution. As her mother describes it, "There is a child's toy, made out of col-orful, soft, foam-like nonallergenic material, composed of pieces that fit together like a puzzle. I got this at Toys R Us. It is about one yard square, and using several of these, we made 'rugs' around her bed. She absolutely loves this—she can write her name with the pieces and play with the shapes."

Marie doesn't vacuum when her child is home, or at least puts her in another room during the process. She doesn't clean the bathroom or kitchen surfaces then either, and when she does clean she uses cleaners that are the most odor free and leaves the window open for ventilation. The family also bought air cleaners with special HEPA filters, which remove dust mites and other allergens. A large one sits in the living room and a smaller one in Alex's bedroom. Because the cleaners are noisy, they keep them on only during the day. When they spend weekends away from home, they always take one of the air cleaners with them.

Maintaining Progress

During this program, Alex's health improved slowly but steadily, and her need for antibiotics and asthma medication has dwindled to almost nothing. During the first year on the program, she still required antibiotics a few times, but this was a far cry from the monthly merry-go-round of ear infections, asthma, and medication. In 1997 she only had one infection that required conventional medication, and she has had no antibiotics at all in 1998.

Her mother says, "She's not getting sick as often, even though here in upstate New York it is cold six months out of the year. Even when she gets a cold, it's usually *just* a cold and she recovers from it quickly. She has had only two asthma flare-ups all winter, and they were mild enough to treat at home with the nebulizer. And I used a minimum amount of medication—only twice a day, morning and night, not every four hours."

As Alex's health improved, her parents were able to ease back on the strict diet, and today she needs to limit only foods to which she is allergic because her system has been so cleared of toxins. They now allow her to have some foods with sugar, yeast, dairy, and additives, for example. "I still keep a watchful eye on the amounts of these things she is eating and find a way to keep her happy. For instance, in the summertime I used to give her only sorbet, which is dairy-free. Now I alternate this with ice cream, which she prefers. I always try to give her a choice. And she accepts this. As a special treat I also give her a little bit of chocolate once a month, if she wants it, and in between we don't eat it in front of her. Fortunately, times have changed and the kids don't get much candy at school these days, so she isn't tempted there, either." Marie still prepares her daughter's school lunch, but only because the school she now attends doesn't provide lunch.

Alex doesn't take her multivitamin anymore, unless her mother notices that she is getting sick again. But she does take vitamin C and calcium every day. They continue to give the herbal formula and expectorant everyday, as a preventive, and use natural remedies for colds and allergies.

Today Alex is four years old and back to her vibrant, healthy self. Her parents couldn't be happier. Looking back, Marie says, "Going on the program was a lot of work, but it was definitely worth it. It asked more of me as a parent; I needed to be more actively involved, and to involve teachers and family. We had to change our habits, especially during the initial period when her immune system was being strengthened. But it's not really a lot more work than conventional treatment, if you think about it. On conventional medicine, she was always getting sick, or we were worried that she would get sick. We were always taking her to the doctor or the emergency room with ear infections or asthma, giving her albuterol and antibiotics. These things have terrible side effects on a two-year-old. She has no unwanted effects from the natural treatments. The first ten months was difficult; she improved very slowly and she still got sick, but eventually she overcame that and got better. As Dr. Bock said, this would not have happened if I had kept her on conventional medicines—after four, five years on drugs she wouldn't have improved, she would only have stayed the same."

JEFFREY

When we first saw Jeffrey he was a very small, pale toddler who was having serious ear infections which we suspected were caused by allergies. By age three he had his first asthma episode, and when we tested him for allergies we found that he was extremely allergic to many inhaled substances, including dust and dust mites, cat dander, and tree and grass pollen.

Although he was highly allergic, Jeffrey was very afraid of needles, so we did not prescribe allergy desensitization shots. Rather, we prescribed a combination of environmental controls, nutritional and herbal supplements, and homeopathic remedies. Getting Jeffrey to follow the plan was not smooth sailing—he was a feisty little guy, finicky about food, revolted by the taste of herbal remedies, and was always asking, "Why do I have to do this?" We had to be flexible and clever and sometimes use humor to ease the way.

Rebecca, his mother, says, "I breast-fed Jeffrey exclusively for the first six months of his life, and he grew beautifully. He weighed sixteen pounds at six months! But when I introduced other food, he stopped thriving and took the next year and a half to add three pounds more.

"One of the nice things about seeing Dr. Bock was that he was treating the whole family. He knew we all have allergies—in fact, I had asthma as a child—and he told us there was a good chance that Jeffrey would have them, too. So I wasn't that surprised when he tested positive for many things. Still, I was frightened when he had his first asthma attack and wanted to do everything I could to get him well."

Cleaning up the Environment

Because Jeffrey had so many allergies, the first thing we did was to recommend that the family work on his environment to minimize his exposure to these potential asthma triggers. For instance, they had two cats in the house, and Jeffrey was highly allergic to their dander. His mother says, "I put the cats in the basement and did not allow them to be upstairs in the house when Jeffrey was

> **JEFFREY'S ASTHMA CONTROL PROGRAM**
>
> - environmental controls (remove cats, HEPA air filter, professional house cleaner, anti–dust mite bedding)
> - modified optimum diet
> - multi-vitamin-mineral supplement
> - vitamin C supplement
> - liquid magnesium
> - flaxseed oil
> - echinacea for colds

home. I saw a big difference from that in just one month. I also bought an air cleaner with a HEPA filter, which sits in his room and is on all day long. That made a difference too. I have a professional come in and thoroughly clean his room every two weeks. I'm really strict about it. If I see one speck of dust she gets a lecture from me.

"Fortunately, I never had carpeting in his room, so I didn't have to deal with that. I started to wash his sheets in hot water every week to get rid of dust mites and ordered a special anti-dust-mite bedding. This also helped reduce his allergic symptoms, but I realized that although I can minimize his exposure to these allergens at home, when he goes to other places, there's always the chance that he will be exposed to a trigger. A good example is elm trees, to which he is very allergic. There are elm trees on the school grounds, as well as at his grandmother's house. In fact, he suffered his first two asthma attacks at his grandmother's house, and there's no way we were going to avoid visiting grandma. So it was clear we had to work to restore his immune system on other levels, too."

Diet and Nutrition

Because Jeffrey was underweight and such a picky eater, we did not push for big changes in his diet. Although we usually recommend a vegetarian or near-vegetarian eating pattern, it was not appropriate in Jeffrey's case.

"Jeffrey couldn't adapt to a vegetarian, or even a semivegetarian diet," says Rebecca. "Unfortunately. But when he was young and so small for his age he was not even on the growth chart, I had to get *something* into the little guy, and what he liked best was things like chopped meat and hot dogs. So I let him have them. Although I didn't restrict his foods, I did try to encourage him to eat fruits and vegetables because Dr. Bock emphasized the fact that they have the nutrients he needed to overcome asthma. Still, I remember there was a period when I couldn't get *any* vegetables into him. It sounds horrendous, but the only way I could get him to eat broccoli was to chop it in the food processor along with some carrots, and sprinkle it with maple syrup and grated cheese. I try to get as many organic foods as possible—even though where we live the organic produce wouldn't win any beauty contests—and avoid buying those foods I know are most likely to be contaminated with pesticides, such as grapes."

His mother's efforts to get him to eat fruits and vegetables was a good start. We felt Jeffrey also needed to add nutrient supplements and herbs to his regimen. To be sure he got a full complement of vitamins and minerals, we recommended he take a full-spectrum, high-potency formula every day. Rebecca buys a children's vegetarian formula at a health food store that is chewable, and, luckily for everyone, Jeffrey likes the taste. She also started giving him vitamin C every day. It's the chewable kind too, and it comes in two flavors that she alternates from day to day so he doesn't burn out on the taste.

We also prescribed flaxseed oil to reduce the chronic inflammation that was causing the asthma. His mother noticed that it also helped alleviate Jeffrey's tendency to constipation, which would be an important step in ridding his body of the toxins that would irritate his system and worsen inflammation. This is an excellent example of how natural therapies can have more than one beneficial effect.

Jeffrey readily accepted these supplements. Not so Chinese herbs! When we tried to get him to take a Chinese herbal formula that was designed to strengthen the lungs, he turned up his nose and refused to take it. Says his mother, "He gave me such a hard time about it that I decided to taste it and I immediately understood why he had made such a fuss—it tasted awful! So I just stopped giving it to him and Dr. Bock moved onto something else."

Next, we tried liquid magnesium, which relaxes the muscles around the airways. This didn't taste that great either, but it wasn't as bad as the herbs and Jeffrey agreed to take it after we had a talk with him about how much better it would make him feel.

Rebecca understood that it was wise to keep all conventional drugs to a minimum. We also wanted to nip any colds in the bud, to avoid triggering asthma. We recommended echinacea tincture as a preventive and treatment. "When I saw a cold coming on, I gave him echinacea tincture," his mother says. "He doesn't like the taste, but I disguise it in orange juice and call it 'Dr. Bock's Special Medicine,' which gets a sly giggle out of Jeffrey. When I start this at the first sign of a cold and continue for five days, he gets over the cold pretty quickly and it doesn't turn into asthma."

Preventive Maintenance

Jeffrey has blossomed into an articulate, self-aware, self-reliant little person. The pale, weak boy is now six years old and of normal height and weight for his age. Rebecca says, "He's really quite healthy now, and maintaining his health requires very little effort. I use conventional asthma medicine only when he needs it, which is rare—twice this year. He sometimes says asthma slows him down, but he's mostly very energetic and active.

"Although he's feisty and challenges everything, now he's old enough so that when I explain why we are doing something, he understands. If I can give him a reason to do something that he can connect with, he does it. For example, I encourage him to drink water all the time. I tell him it is good for keeping the mucus liquid and flowing and also for his constipation. Today, he eats vegetables without my having to disguise them with maple syrup and cheese because he knows they are good for him and he needs them to be strong for his Tai Kwan Do."

Jeffrey has learned to monitor his own symptoms and to take care of himself. His mother is proud that "If he starts to have symptoms and gets short of breath, he knows that's when it's time to slow down a little bit, to drink water." This most often occurs in the spring, when there's pollen in the air, and he's running around with all the natural exuberance of childhood. "It's amazing to me how quickly he was able to take charge of his own care," says his mother. "If I forget to put the vitamins out in the morning, he reminds me!" He still gets liquid magnesium occasionally, when his parents notice the early signs of an asthma flare-up. He only needs it for a week or two, until the wheezing stops. And they continue to give him echinacea if they see a cold coming on.

"It really wasn't difficult making these changes and understanding why they were needed. Maybe it was so natural and easy for us to follow the program because my parents have always been into vitamin therapy—all of us kids used to take cod liver oil regularly, and my mother put raw garlic in our salads, and gave us an extra clove in the morning during flu season before we went off to school. We started taking vitamin supplements when we were twelve years old." Clearly, Rebecca's upbringing made it easier psychologically to fit the Natural Asthma Control Program into her family's life. But her son's condition and personality required more—ingenuity, persistence, and a flexible attitude—to give her story a happy ending.

CAITLIN

When we first saw Caitlin she was only five years old, yet she had already been diagnosed with asthma and recurrent sinusitis and bronchitis. She also suffered from a constant cough, allergies, and frequent bouts of the "croup." Her tiny body had been wracked by respiratory infections all winter, and she was being treated with a slew of medications for asthma and allergic rhinitis, and had been on and off antibiotics for most of her young life. Under a conventional allergist's care, Caitlin only got worse and suffered a vaginal yeast infection due to overuse of antibiotics. When we tested her to find specific allergens, we discovered many allergies her allergist had missed. We put her on a hypoallergenic diet that was also antiyeast and began treatment with antiyeast medication. Nutritional supplements and avoiding as many environmental allergens as possible helped as well. However, since her family was unable to avoid mold, we decided to add a special immunotherapy desensitization technique. When we added these injections to all the other measures, her health improved even more, and Caitlin can live a more normal life and even have her dog around again most of the time.

Caitlin's mother, Kim, tells of her fear and frustration during her daughter's darkest moments. "She would cough and cough and cough all night, and this of course ruined her sleep—and ours. There was nothing I could do to help her. I tried honey, cough drops, cough medicine—nothing worked. When she was around four years old, I took her to a conventional allergist. He was the first to diagnose her with asthma. Her father and I were extremely upset and alarmed when we heard this. The allergist had tested her for allergies and advised us to remove as many allergens as possible from our home. So, we tore through the house, ripping out the wall-to-wall carpeting in her room and replacing it with a different floor, putting away all her stuffed animals in the attic, installing air conditioning. We kept the dog outside—that was really difficult because my husband and I got her before we were married, and she was like a family member. We cleaned and cleaned and used special vacuum cleaners. Now that I look back on it, I think I might have cleaned too much, with harsh chemical cleansers that may have contributed to Caitlin's allergies.

"All the allergist did by way of treatment was to give her more drugs. He prescribed inhaler steroids—he wanted her to take them three times a day, even when she didn't have symptoms. I didn't like this idea, but I didn't know what else to do, so we continued with this doctor for a year. However, it seemed like every time we turned around we were taking her back to the doctor for more antibiotics. And the more drugs we were putting into her, the sicker she was getting. Each time it was worse than the time before—she'd cough so bad in the middle of the night, we'd rush to her bedroom, and her lips would be blue, she'd look at me, totally petrified and miserable, and she couldn't even cry because she couldn't breathe. One time she was so sick she brought up blood clots. We were panic-stricken, and I knew we were heading towards a time when she would be so sick, we'd have to take her to the emergency room. Then I found Dr. Bock, through someone

I knew at work. Through his integrative approach, we were able to completely turn her health around."

An Integrated Approach

When we tested Caitlin at our health center, we discovered she had many food allergies. She also had an overgrowth of yeast in her body. Her mother says, "When I found out about Caitlin's food allergies I was so angry. I confronted my previous doctor and asked why he didn't tell me about them, about the yeast problem. He just got defensive and said natural medicine was controversial. I said, 'But this stuff is working—yours was not!'"

Caitlin's parents needed to restrict her diet quite a bit. Like Alex's mother, Kim was dismayed when she started reading food labels. "Caitlin had to avoid dairy, yeast, and sugar, and these are in everything—it was overwhelming, a real eye-opener. I had to start shopping at health food stores to find breads with no yeast or sugar. I gave her special lunches, but this set her apart from the other kids, and she was embarrassed to eat her food at school, I'm sorry to say. It was hard. One day she came home from school with chocolate all over her face. I asked her if she had eaten chocolate. She looked me straight in the eye and said 'no.' This happened more than once."

CAITLIN'S ASTHMA CONTROL PROGRAM

- environmental controls (no wall-to-wall carpeting, remove stuffed animals, air conditioning, dog lives outside, HEPA vacuum cleaner)
- hypoallergenic diet
- multi-vitamin-mineral supplement
- vitamin C supplement, plus bioflavonoids
- calcium supplement
- acidophilus
- borage oil
- Chinese herbal tonic
- EPD desensitization shots

In addition to changing her diet, Kim gave Caitlin a variety of nutritional supplements to boost her immune system, control the yeast overgrowth, and dampen the inflammatory process. She takes a multi-vitamin-mineral formula with extra calcium because she eats no dairy, and extra vitamins E and C with bioflavonoids. She also gets acidophilus ("beneficial" bacteria to restore intestinal health), borage oil for essential fatty acids, and a Chinese herbal formula containing astragalus as a tonic to strengthen her resistance to infection.

One thing that the family was not able to change significantly is the presence of mold. They live in a house situated in a low-lying area, surrounded by streams, moisture, and bushes. In short, the perfect place for mold to flourish. We felt that since both Caitlin and her mother had allergies, they needed to be high and dry, not low and wet, because we suspected that mold was acting as a potent trigger. Indeed, her parents noticed that when they visited her grandmother's house, which was situated higher up, Caitlin felt better. This seemed to support our theory that mold was a problem, but the family was not about to move to another location because they had designed and built their beloved house themselves.

Although mold was an ongoing presence in the house, Caitlin was improving under the program. Still, we felt that under the circumstances, more should be done to further enhance the recovery of this very sick little girl. We suggested special desensitization shots called EPD (explained on page 49), for mold, certain foods, and animal dander. "I must say the shots that Dr. Bock gave her have helped tremendously," enthuses her mother. "They've changed our lives. She got them for a total of about a year and a half. She's much less sensitive to the mold in the house and to foods. The dog can live in the house in the winter, and when Caitlin starts sneezing, I just move the dog to another room."

Today

"Caitlin is doing really well," says Kim. "Before we started this program she had been on antibiotics pretty much all the time, and now I can't recall the last time she took antibiotics. She has used her asthma reliever medicine only once in the last year." But it still isn't totally smooth sailing.

"When she was younger, she was more cooperative," observes her mother. "But now she is eight years old and sometimes she's not so good about taking the pills. One thing I notice that helps is that if I can make sure that she eats enough, at least the pills don't give her an upset stomach. But as she's getting older, she is asking me more and more, 'Why do I have to do this?' I tell her it's because it makes her feel better, but it's hard for her to remember how sick she was. She just wants to go about living her active, happy life as a normal child. I wonder what will happen when she becomes a teenager, and she starts to rebel even more?

"If there's one thing I want to say to other parents, it's this: You've got to have an open mind. Educate yourself, read everything you can get your hands on. Talk to other parents of children with asthma—you'd be surprised how much they can teach you, especially about practical things like getting your child to eat better. This program is work, but it's worth it. I never think it's too much of a bother, too much work. My daughter is my whole life. I want her to be healthy and to have a good life, to not think of herself as sick. And only an integrated approach has been able to give her that."

As these families demonstrate, using our Natural Asthma Control Program to combine natural therapies with conventional therapies gives you a way to provide the absolute best care for your child. We hope that you will use this book to take the opportunity to play a more active role in assuming responsibility for your child's condition. It takes effort at first—less, as time goes by—and in the process, you are accomplishing much more than asthma control. You are encouraging an independence of relying on drugs as a quick fix. And, just as important, you are laying the foundations of good physical and emotional health, giving your child the gift of a strong constitution that will help him or her resist other serious conditions. In short, you are giving your child the normal, healthy life that is every child's birthright.

GLOSSARY

Acupuncture—A technique used in traditional Chinese medicine which punctures the skin with thin needles at certain points of the body in order to manipulate the chi, or life force. In acupressure, no needles are used; rather, fingers are used to press the points.

Adrenaline—A hormone released during times of stress by the adrenal glands that can relax bronchial tubes; also known as epinephrine.

Airflow limitation—A term used to describe an exhalation that takes longer than four seconds due to asthma. This term is preferred over the customary phrases "airway obstruction" and "airway narrowing," which imply specific mechanisms of airflow limitation, because there are several possible mechanisms.

Airway hyperresponsiveness—Airways that narrow too easily or too much in response to a provoking stimulus; also called hypersensitivity or hyperreactivity. In asthma, airways can be hyperresponsive to many different stimuli.

Allergen—A substance that causes an allergic reaction. Common allergens are dust, pollen, animal dander, and chemicals in air, water, and food.

Allergy—A condition in which the immune system responds in an inappropriate or exaggerated way to certain substances that are harmless or even useful. This response does not occur in nonallergic individuals who are exposed to the same substance.

Allopathic medicine—A system of medicine that often entails suppressing the symptoms, rather than supporting the body's innate ability to heal. Also called conventional or mainstream medicine.

Alveoli—The tiny air sacs in the lungs where oxygen and carbon dioxide are exchanged between the blood and air.

Antibody—A protein produced by the white blood cells called lymphocytes in response to an allergen or other foreign body such as a virus. Antibody is also known as immunoglobulin. Bacteria, viruses, and other microorganisms commonly contain many antigens, as do pollens, dust mites, molds, foods, and other substances. Although many types of antibodies are protective, inappropriate or excessive formation of antibodies may lead to illness. When the body forms a type of antibody called IgE (immunoglobulin E), allergic rhinitis, asthma, or eczema may result when the patient is again exposed to the substance that caused IgE antibody formation (allergen).

Antigen—A substance that stimulates the immune system to produce antibodies to protect the body. An allergen is a special type of antigen which causes an IgE antibody response.

Antihistamine—A substance that reduces the effects of histamine, a chemical made by the body in response to a foreign substance (allergen).

Anti-inflammatory—A substance, such as a nutrient, herb, or drug that inhibits one or more of the components of the inflammatory reaction.

Antioxidant—A molecule made by the body or eaten as a food or supplement which chemically prevents oxidation of cells by free radicals.

Asthma—A chronic lung condition resulting from bronchial tubes obstructed because of muscle constriction, excess mucus, or swelling and inflammation.

Atopic asthma—Asthma due to an inherited allergy; often associated with atopic eczema, a skin condition. Atopy is the propensity, usually genetic, for developing immune responses involving immunoglobulin E (IgE) to common environmental allergens.

Autonomic nervous system—The part of the nervous system that controls involuntary body functions including breathing and heartbeat.

B-cells—White blood cells of the immune system that are produced in the bone marrow and produce antibodies.

Botanicals—Medicines derived from plants, including herbs.

Bronchi—The large tube-like air passages through which air moves to and from the lungs; also called bronchial tubes.

Bronchioles—The small air passages that branch off from the bronchi.

Bronchitis—Inflammation of the mucus membranes of the lungs, resulting in a persistent cough and production of phlegm.

Bronchodilator—A substance used to open up the air passages to prevent and treat asthma symptoms.

Bronchoconstriction—Airflow limitation due to contraction of airway smooth muscle. "Bronchoconstriction" is preferred to the word "bronchospasm."

Bronchodilator drugs—Drugs that widen the airways in the lungs by allowing the muscles surrounding them to relax.

Cilia—Tiny hairs lining the respiratory tract which sweep mucus, pollen, dust, viruses, and other particles out of the air passages.

Complement—Protein molecules released when an antibody locks onto an antigen and penetrates the outer shell of the foreign body.

Controller medications—Medications taken daily on a long-term basis that are useful in getting persistent asthma under control and in maintaining control. They include anti-inflammatory agents such as corticosteroids and long-acting bronchodilators. Controller medications are also sometimes called prophylactic, preventive, regular preventive, or maintenance medications.

Corticosteroids—Drugs that reduce inflammation of bronchial passages because they are similar hormones produced by the cortex of the adrenal gland.

Cyanosis—A blue tinge of the lips, nails, and skin caused by a deficiency of oxygen and an excess of carbon dioxide in the blood; this may occur during a severe asthma attack.

Dander—Microscopic scales from the skin, feathers, or fur of animals, which can cause allergic reaction in people.

Decoction—A strong brew of herb tea made by boiling and then steeping the roots and bark in water.

Dyspnea—Labored or difficult breathing caused by "air hunger" during a moderate to severe asthma attack.

Extract—A concentrated herbal preparation made with water.

Extrinsic asthma—Asthma that is triggered by exposure to allergens.

Flavonoids (Bioflavonoids)—A group of chemicals found in plants that are helpful in many essential body functions, including protection from free radicals.

Free radical—An unstable molecule lacking an electron which steals an electron from other molecules in cells of the body, thus harming the cells, including those of the immune system.

Guided imagery—A form of self-therapy in which a person creates an image in his or her mind of a desired outcome, such as white cells destroying a virus.

Helper T-cells—White blood cells that patrol the blood stream and recognize antigens and alert other components of the immune system.

Histamine—A compound that mast cells release as part of the immune response to a foreign body to protect the body from allergens; this allergic reaction causes inflammation, increased blood flow, and mucus production. During an asthma episode, it is responsible for narrowing the bronchi or airways in the lungs.

Homeopathy—A system of medicine based on the principle of "like cures like"; it treats a person by administering a very small dose of a medication that would bring on the symptoms of the disease if taken by a healthy person.

Hyperreactive airways—Airways that are more sensitive than normal and that overreact to a stimulus, often causing tightening or narrowing.

Hyperventilation—Faster or deeper breathing that creates an excess intake of oxygen and results in lightheadedness, dizziness, and chest pain.

Immune system—A complex system of cells and proteins that protects the body from infection of potentially harmful, infectious microorganisms (microscopic life-forms), such as bacteria, viruses, and fungi. This system consists of the various types of white blood cells and the lymphatic system, which includes the thymus gland, lymph tissues, and spleen. The immune system also plays a role in the control of cancer and other diseases, but also is involved in allergies, hypersensitivity, and asthma.

Immunoglobulins—Five distinct antibodies formed in response to certain antigens; with asthma, an excess of immunoglobulin E (IgE) is produced, and this results in an allergic reaction.

Influenza—A highly contagious viral infection of the upper respiratory tract that may be serious.

Infusion—The most common method of preparing herb tea,

made by pouring boiling water over the petals, flowers, or
leaves and allowing it to steep.

Inhaler—An aerosol device used to give medication to a
patient's lungs while a patient breathes in.

Interferon—A protein released by cells that are under attack
by viruses and which protects neighboring cells from
infection.

Interleukin 1—A protein of the immune system that activates T-cells and macrophages and causes inflammation
and fever.

Intrinsic asthma—Asthma that is not related to allergic reaction; rather it is associated with other respiratory problems such as infection.

Leukocytes—White blood cells.

Lymphocytes—T-cells and B-cells that arise from the lymph
glands; they are usually about 25 percent of the total
white cell count but increase in number when there is an
infection.

Macrophages—Large white blood cells that patrol the body
and that surround and digest foreign substances such as
viruses.

Mast cells—Large cells that are located throughout the body,
including the bronchi, that release substances including
histamine.

Mites—Microscopic insects that exist in house dust, human
and animal skin, and feathers; they collect in mattresses,
bedcovers, and carpets and can cause allergic reaction in
some people.

Mold—A type of fungus that produces microscopic spores
that can cause an allergic reaction in some people when
inhaled.

Mucosa—Mucous membranes that line the inside surface of
the mouth, throat, and nose and contain mucus glands.

Mucus—A sticky body fluid produced by the mucus glands that coats, moistens, and protects the membranes.

Natural killer cells—T-cells that attack and destroy viruses and other harmful particles, including cancer cells.

Naturopathic medicine—A form of natural healing that treats the whole person, including the mind, body, and spirit.

Nebulizer—A device that turns liquid medicine into a mist which is easy for children to inhale through a mask.

Peak flow meter—A self-diagnostic device that people with asthma blow into in order to measure the strength of their exhalation and thus help monitor the condition of their lungs and give early warning of an impending attack.

Phagocytes—White blood cells that scavenge and mop up debris after other immune system components have done their job.

Phytochemicals or phytonutrients—A group of chemicals contained in plant foods (fruits, vegetables, herbs) that have a beneficial effect on health; phytochemicals and their functions are still being discovered.

Pollen—Microscopic spores from plants that can cause an allergic reaction in some people when inhaled.

Prostaglandins—Hormone-like fatty acids that have a variety of functions, including inflammation.

Receptor—A "docking site" on the surface of a cell that receives a chemical and passes a message into the cell.

Rhinovirus—The type of virus that causes most colds; there are over two hundred varieties.

Reliever medications—Short-acting bronchodilating medications that act quickly to relieve airflow limitation and its accompanying acute symptoms such as cough, chest tightness, and wheezing. Relievers are also sometimes called "quick relief medicine" or "rescue medicine."

Spacer—A device that helps children get asthma medicine

into the lungs by first dispensing the medication into a chamber from which they can inhale it more slowly.

Spirometer—An instrument used in pulmonary function tests to measure the amount and speed of the air moving in and out of the lungs.

Suppressor T-cells—White blood cells that wind down the immune response after it has dealt with an infection.

T-cells—White blood cells made in the bone marrow that mature in the thymus gland.

Tincture—A concentrated herbal preparation made with alcohol.

Wheezing—A high-pitched hissing or whistling sound caused by difficulty breathing out.

Zone system—A system used to manage asthma, based on specified levels of symptoms and peak expiratory flow measured with a peak flow meter. Typically, the system resembles that of a traffic light, with green (all clear), yellow (caution), and red (danger) zones. This approach helps patients monitor their disease, identify the earliest possible signs that the day-to-day control of asthma is deteriorating, and act quickly to regain control. In conventional medicine, this type of system guides you in using medications, environmental control measures, and contact with a health care professional for each zone. In this book, we use it also to guide you in using natural therapies.

REFERENCE NOTES

"Asthma and Oxidant Stress: Nutritional, Environmental, and Genetic Factors." *Journal of the American College of Nutrition* 14, no. 4 (Aug 1995): 317–24.

"Asthma and Vitamin C." *Environment & Health News* 1, no. 3: 10.

"Asthmatic Children Particularly Vulnerable to Outdoor Air Pollution." *American Journal of Respiratory and Critical Care Medicine* 157 (1998): 1034–43.

Brody, Jane. "Steroids Interfere with Both Calcium and Hormones." *New York Times*, 14 May 1997.

"Certain Asthma Medications Contain Bronchoconstricting Preservative." *Pharmacotherapy* 18 (1998): 130–139.

"Fish Oils Help Asthma." *International Journal of Alternative and Complementary Medicine* 15, no. 5 (May 1996): 7.

"Inhaled and Nasal Glucocorticoids and the Risks of Ocular Hypertension or Open-angle Glaucoma." *Journal of the American Medical Association* 277 (March 5, 1997): 722–27.

Kleinman, Ronald. "Parents May Know Correct Answers, but Don't Implement Proper Nutrition." Presentation at the American Medical Association media briefing on nutrition, September 18, 1997.

"Magnesium and Bronchial Asthma." *International Journal of Alternative and Complementary Medicine* (February 1996): 14.

"Many U.S. Medical Schools Offer Alternative Medicine Courses." *Journal of the American Medical Association*, 280 (1998): 784–87.

Redd, Stephen. "Asthma Rising Dramatically in the United States." Presentation at an American Medical Association media briefing on advances in treating and managing asthma, May 7, 1998.

"Regular Bronchodilators Worsen Asthma Control." *The Lancet* 336 (1990): 1391.

Sampson, Hugh A. "Number of People with Food Allergies on the Rise." Presentation at the American Medical Association media briefing on nutrition, September 18, 1997.

"Use of Inhaled Corticosteroids and the Risk of Cataracts." *The New England Journal of Medicine* 337, no.1 (July 3, 1997).

"Vegan Regimen with Reduced Medication in the Treatment of Bronchial Asthma." *Journal of Asthma* 22, no. 44 (1985): 13.

"Wheeze May Not Reflect Asthma Severity." *Health Psychology* 16, no. 6 (1997): 547–53.

"Bedroom Cockroach Allergen Levels Tied to Sensitivity in Asthmatic Children." *Journal of Allergy and Clinical Immunology* (1998); 102: 536–570.

RESOURCES

SUGGESTED READING LIST

You may be able to find these books at your local bookstore; if not, they can order them for you. Alternatively, you can order them via the Internet through Amazon or Barnes and Noble. These two large on-line bookstores carry a wide selection of books on asthma, often at discounted prices. Amazon has the added feature of providing short summaries and comments by readers.

Amazon
www.amazon.com
fax: 206-694-2950
phone: 800-201-7575 for U.S. customers or 206-694-2992 for international customers.

Barnes and Noble
www.barnesandnoble.com

Books about Natural Healing

Bauer, Cathryn. *Acupressure for Everybody.* New York: Henry Holt, 1991.

Bock, Kenneth, and Nellie Sabin. *The Road to Immunity.* New York, Pocket Books, 1997.

Brown, Donald. *Herbal Prescriptions for Better Health.* Rocklin, Calif.: Prima Publishing, 1996.

Bruning, Nancy and Corey Weinstein, M.D. *Healing Homeopathic Remedies*. New York: Dell Publishing, 1996.

Castleman, Michael. *Nature's Cures*. Emmaus, Penn.: Rodale Press, 1996.

Castleman, Michael. *The Healing Herbs*. Emmaus, Penn.: Rodale Press, 1991.

Castro, Miranda. *The Complete Homeopathy Handbook*. New York: St. Martin's Press, 1990.

Colbin, Annemarie. *Food and Healing*. New York: Ballantine, 1986.

Cummings, Stephen, and Dana Ullman. *Everybody's Guide to Homeopathic Medicines: Taking Care of Yourself and Your Family with Safe and Effective Remedies*. Los Angeles: J.P. Tarcher, 1991.

Elias, Jason. *The A-to-Z Guide to Healing Herbal Remedies*. New York: Dell Publishing, 1995.

Fezler, William. *Total Visualization: Using All Five Senses*. Englewood Cliffs, N.J.: Prentice-Hall, 1992.

Ford, Norman D. *Eighteen Natural Ways to Beat the Common Cold*. New Canaan, Conn.: Keats Publishing, 1987.

Gach, Michael Reed. *Acupressure's Potent Points*. New York: Bantam Books, 1990.

Hendler, Sheldon Saul. *The Doctor's Vitamin and Mineral Encyclopedia*. New York: Fireside/Simon and Schuster, 1990.

Krieger, Delores. *Accepting Your Power to Heal: The Personal Practice of Therapeutic Touch*. Santa Fe, N.M.: Bear, 1993.

Lappe, Marc. *When Antibiotics Fail: Restoring the Ecology of the Body*. Berkeley, Calif.: North Atlantic Books, 1995.

Lieberman, Shari, and Nancy Bruning. *The Real Vitamin & Mineral Book*. 2d ed. Garden City Park, N.Y.: Avery Publishing Group, 1997.

Mindell, Earl. *Earl Mindells' Herb Bible.* New York: Simon and Schuster, 1992.

Murray, Michael. *The Healing Power of Herbs.* 2d ed. Rocklin, Calif.: Prima Publishing, 1995.

Namikoshi, Toru. *The Complete Book of Shiatsu Therapy.* Tokyo and New York: Japan Publications, 1981.

Pearsall, Paul. *The Pleasure Prescription: To Love, to Work, to Play—Life in the Balance.* Alameda, Calif.: Hunter House, 1996.

Tierra, Michael. *The Way of Herbs.* New York: Pocket Books, 1990.

Weil, Andrew. *Natural Health, Natural Healing.* Boston: Houghton-Mifflin, 1990.

Books about Asthma and Allergies

Altman, Nathaniel. *What You Can Do About Asthma.* New York: Dell Publishing, 1991.

The American Lung Association Asthma Advisory Group. *Family Guide to Asthma and Allergies.* New York: Little, Brown and Company, 1997.

Bower, John and Lynn. *The Healthy House: How to Buy One, How to Build One, How to Cure a "Sick" One.* Bloomington, Ill.: Healthy House Institute, 1997.

Buchanan, Neil, and Peter Cooper. *Childhood Asthma: What It Is and What You Can Do.* Berkeley, Calif.: Tricycle Press, 1991.

Cutler, Ellen. *Winning the War Against Asthma & Allergies.* Albany, N.Y.: Delmar Publishers, 1997.

Firshein, Richard. *Reversing Asthma: Reduce Your Medications with this Revolutionary New Program.* New York: Warner Books, 1996.

Haas, Francois, and Shiela Sperber Haas. *The Essential Asthma Book: A Manual for Asthmatics of All Ages.* New York: Ivy Books, 1987.

Hamilton, Kirk R. and Kristine A. Roberson. *Asthma: Clinical Pearls in Nutrition and Complementary Therapies.* IT Services, 1997 (hard to find, available through Amazon.com).

Klein, Gerald, and Vicki Timerman. *Keys to Parenting the Asthmatic Child.* Hauppauge, N.Y.: Barron's Educational Series, 1994.

The Natural Medicine Collective with Gary McLain. *The Natural Way of Healing Asthma and Allergies.* New York: Dell Publishing, 1995.

Plaut, Thomas. *Children with Asthma: A Manual for Parents.* Amherst, Mass.: Pedipress, Inc., 1995.

Polk, Irwin. *All About Asthma.* New York: Plenum Press, 1997.

Potterton, David. *All About Asthma and Its Treatment without Drugs.* London: Foulsham Publishing House, 1995.

Pressman, Alan, and Herbert Goodman. *Treating Asthma, Allergies and Food Sensitivities.* New York: Berkeley Books, 1997.

Puotinen, C.J. *Herbs to Help You Breathe Freely.* New Canaan, Conn.: Keats Publishing, Inc., 1994.

Ridgeway, Roy. *The Natural Way with Asthma.* Rockport, Mass.: Element Books, Inc., 1994.

Roberts, Ron, and Judy Sammut. *Asthma: An Alternative Approach.* New Canaan, Conn.: Keats Publishing, Inc. 1997.

Sander, Nancy. *A Parent's Guide to Asthma: How You Can Help Your Child Control Asthma at Home, School, and Play.* New York: Penguin Books, 1994.

Weinstein, Allan M. *Asthma: The Complete Guide to Self-Management of Asthma and Allergies for Patients and Their Families.* New York: Fawcett Crest, 1987.

Weiss, Jonathan. *Breathe Easy: Young People's Guide to Asthma.* New York: Magination Press, 1994.

White, Celeste. *Natural Asthma and Allergy Management.* Redding, Calif.: Keswick House, 1997.

Pedipress, Inc.
125 Red Gate Lane
Amherst, MA 01002
Call 800-611-6081 or 413-549-7798 for credit card orders or shipping outside the forty-eight contiguous states.

Educational materials and monitoring tools covering conventional medicine. Many in English and Spanish, including *Children with Asthma* (manual for parents), *One Minute Asthma* (forty-eight-page basic guide geared towards keeping adults and children out of emergency rooms), Peak Flow Diary (pad of 100 sheets), Signs Diary (pad of 50 sheets).

BOOKS, VIDEOS, AND WEB SITES FOR CHILDREN

Check the Internet for more sources of asthma-related books, information, support, and interactive activities such as games and quizzes.

We are the medical directors of a Web site called PatientsAmerica, which provides education and patient advocacy services. PatientsAmerica also provides a catalog of daily medical tracking forms on a number of illnesses and medical conditions including asthma. These forms are for use by patients, their families, and other caregivers to maintain a daily record of the patient's progress, medications, diet, and other pertinent information. Visitors to the Web site at www.PatientsAmerica.com can review or download the tracking form of their choice, free of charge.

Wheeze World (a take-off on *Wayne's World*), *Free to Breathe* (an entertaining primer), *So You Have Asthma Too* (for preschoolers) are available from Allergy and Asthma Network, see address below. This organization also sells videos for adults, including *Managing Childhood Asthma*.

Bronkie the Bronkiosaurus is a video game that teaches kids how to manage their asthma while maneuvering a dinosaur through a prehistoric environment. Available from Raya Systems, 419-949-3933.

Bergman, Thomas. *Determined to Win: Children Living with Allergies and Asthma*. Milwaukee: Gareth Stevens Publishing, 1994.

Carter, Alden R., and Siri M. Carter. *I'm Tougher Than Asthma!* Morton Grove, Ill: Albert Whitman & Co., 1996. A photo book written by a little girl with asthma.

Dolan, Eileen. *Winning Over Asthma*. 2d ed. Amherst, Mass.: Pedipress, 1996. A thirty-two-page illustrated book that children can use as a coloring book.

Harrington, Geri. *Jackie Joyner-Kersee: Champion Athlete*. New York: Chelsea House, 1995. Part of the series Great Achievers: Lives of the Physically Challenged.

London, Jonathan. *The Lion Who Had Asthma*. Morton Grove, Ill.: Albert Whitman & Co., 1992.

The Asthma and Allergy Foundation of America (AAFA) also publishes materials (see address, below). They include:

• *You Can Control Asthma*—A versatile, user-friendly asthma education tool; makes asthma management a family activity. One of the workbooks is an illustrated "easy reader" book for parents. The companion activity book is for children ages six to twelve.

• *Asthma Care Training for Kids (ACT)*—When kids and their families understand asthma, its triggers, warning signs, and treatment, it is easier to control. ACT's development team—including nurses, physicians and educators—designed the program to help parents and health professionals work with children to manage their asthma.

• *Meeting-in-a-Box*—A self-contained, comprehensive kit with all the components needed for a successful asthma presentation.

• *Power Breathing*—The first asthma education program designed specifically for teens. This hands-on program is characterized by interactive instruction, discussion, and strategic thinking; video animation.

• *Class Dismissed!*—A dynamic board game used to test asthma knowledge.

• *Asthma Challenge*—A question/answer format, team game designed with AAFA Bucks awarded for correct answers. Categories include: "Tools of the Trade," "Sneezes, Wheezes and Triggers Too," and "Nuts and Bolts."

SOURCES FOR ALLERGY-CONTROL PRODUCTS

Contact one or more of the following organizations and mail-order companies for more information about household products and procedures for allergy-proofing your home.

Allergy Control Products
96 Danbury Road
Ridgefield CT 06877
800-422-DUST

Allergy Resources
Box 444
Guffey, CO 80820
800-USE-FLAX

Self-Care
104 Challenger Drive
Portland, TN 37148-1716
800-345-3371

American Academy of Environmental Medicine
4510 W. 89th Street, Suite 110
Prairie Village, KS 66207-2282
913-642-6062

EDUCATIONAL AND
SUPPORT ORGANIZATIONS

For more information, support, educational programs, referral to physicians, practitioners, and other services, contact the following organizations.

Asthma Organizations

Allergy and Asthma Network/Mothers of Asthmatics, Inc. (AAN/MA)
2751 Prosperity Avenue, Suite 150
Fairfax, VA 22031
Toll free: 800-878-4403
Phone: 703-641-9595
Fax: 703-573-7794
e-mail: aanma@aol.com
http://www.aanma.org/
> Provides support for parents of children with asthma; publishes a newsletter and annual resource listing of summer camps and supplies. Books, videos, and other materials for children and adults. Peak flow meters and nebulizer accessories for purchase at reduced cost. Maintains toll-free hotline answered by trained staff. Monthly newsletter with AAN/MA membership.

American Academy of Allergy, Asthma and Immunology
(AAAAI)
611 East Wells Street
Milwaukee, WI 53202
Phone: 800-842-7777
414-272-6071
Fax: 414-276-3349
http://www.aaaai.org/
> The toll-free number listed above can be used for board-certified physician referral and information. Brochures, booklets, newsletters, and videos available.

American Academy of Pediatrics (AAP)
141 North West Point Boulevard
Elk Grove Village, IL 60007
Phone: 847-228-5008
Fax: 847-228-7035
http://www.aap.org
> Brochures on asthma/allergy.

American College of Allergy and Immunology (ACAI)
85 West Algonquin Road, Suite 350
Arlington Heights, IL 60005-4422
Phone: 847-427-1200
800-842-7777
Fax: 874-427-1294
http://allergy.mcg.edu
> Booklets and other materials on allergies and asthma. Most information in booklets and other materials appears on the Web site. Toll-free number for booklets and materials on asthma. Toll-free number for list of allergists by state.

American College of Chest Physicians (ACCP)
3300 Dundee Road
Northbrook, IL 60062
Phone: 847-498-1400
800-343-ACCP
Fax: 847-498-5450
http:www.chestnet.org/
  Toll-free number for brochure on asthma. Look for the
  Chicago Asthma Consortium section on the ACCP Web
  site.

American Lung Association (ALA)
Main office:
1740 Broadway
New York, NY 10010
212-315-8748
e-mail: ala@aol.com
http://www.lungusa.org
  More than one-hundred-sixty print materials available
  on lung health; also provides lists of summer camps for
  children with asthma. Contact local chapters for information and pamphlets. For printed materials, call 1-800-
  LUNG USA or 1-800-586-4872.

Asthma and Allergy Foundation of America (AAFA)
1125 15th Street N.W., Suite 502
Washington, DC 20005
202-466-7643; 800-7-ASTHMA
Fax: 202-466-8940
http://www.aafa.org
  Clearinghouse for information about new treatments for
  asthma. Current and affordable educational pamphlets,

books and other materials on asthma and allergies, with special emphasis on material for children and teens. Videos and educational interactive CD-ROM games for children available. Sponsors a nationwide network of affiliated AAFA chapters. Resource list and prices available upon request. Bimonthly newsletter with AAFA membership.

Asthmatic Children's Foundation
15 Spring Valley Road
Ossining, NY 10562
> Provides treatment and rehabilitation for children with severe asthma.

The National Asthma Education and Prevention Program
National Heart, Lung, and Blood Institute Information Center
P.O. Box 30105
Bethesda, MD 20824-0105
301-251-1222

The National Foundation for Asthma, Inc.
P.O. Box 30069
Tucson, AZ 85751
> Provides health services for children with asthma, particularly when there is financial need.

National Heart, Lung and Blood Institute (NHLBI)
National Institutes of Health
P.O. Box 30105
Bethesda, MD 20824-0105
Phone: 301-251-1222
Fax: 301-251-1223
http://www.nhlbi.nih.gov/nhlbi/nhlbi.htm
> Fact sheets and booklets on controlling asthma and self-management of asthma. Provides listing of asthma publi-

cations and resources, has several educational programs including special publications and materials on asthma for school administrators and school health care workers.

National Jewish Medical and Research Center
1400 Jackson Street
Denver, CO 80206
Phone: 303-388-4461
800-222-LUNG
http://www.njc.org
> The toll-free number can be used to talk to a nurse about problems with asthma or for automated information. Over a dozen booklets on understanding asthma and allergy available.

Support Groups/Chat Rooms/Bulletin Boards

On-Line Living with Asthma Support Group:
www.thriveonline.com/health/asthma/seek/info.selfcare.html

NATURAL MEDICINE:
ORGANIZATIONS AND SUPPLIERS

The American College for Advancement in Medicine
(ACAM)
23121 Verdugo Drive
Suite 204
Laguna Hills, CA 92653
acam@acam.org

American Association of Naturopathic Physicians
2366 Eastlake Ave., East Suite 322
Seattle, WA 98102
206-323-7610 or 206-827-6035
Send $5 for a brochure and list of doctors.

American Holistic Medical Association (AHMA)
6728 Old McLean Village Drive
McLean, VA 22101
703-556-9728; 703-556-9245
   Send $10 for a member directory.

American Academy of Environmental Medicine
P.O. Box 16106
Denver, CO 80216
303-622-9755

Herb Organizations

The American Botanical Council
P.O. Box 201660
Austin, TX 78720
800-373-7105 for catalog
512-331-8868
http://www.herbalgram.org

The American Herbalists Guild
P.O. Box 746555
Arvada, CO 80006
303-423-8800

Herb Research Foundation
1007 Pearl St., Suite 200
Boulder, CO 80302
303-449-2265
800-307-6267 orders only
http://www.herbs.org

Herb and Nutritional Supplement Suppliers

Herbal products are available at health food stores, pharmacies, and herb stores. The following have a reputation for high-quality products; write or phone for information about your nearest distributor or about ordering herbs by mail.

East-West Herb Products
65 Mechanic Street, Suite 103
Red Bank, NJ 07701

East Earth Trade Winds
P.O. Box 493151
Redding, CA 96049
916-223-2346
800-258-6878 for catalog
http://www.snowcrest.net/eetw/
    Chinese herbal formulas.

Eclectic Institute, Inc.
14385 S.E. Lusted Road
Sandy, OR 97055
503-668-4120 (in Oregon); 800-332-4372
www.eclecticherb.com
    Organic herbs.

Herb-Pharm
P.O. Box 116
Williams, OR 97544

Herbs for Kids
151 Evergreen Dr. Suite D
Bozeman, MT 59715
Phone: 406-587-0180
Fax: 406-587-0111
herbs@herbsforkids.com
    Certified organic and pesticide- and alcohol-free herbs
    formulated for children.

Nature's Herb Company
Box 118, Dept. 34,Q
Norway, IA 52318
800-237-0869

Planetary Formulas
P.O. Box 533W
Soquel, CA 95073
800-606-6226

Rainbow Light
207 McPherson St., Dept. P
Santa Cruz, CA 95060
888-669-7766

Rhinebeck Health Nutrients
108 Montgomery Street
Rhinebeck, NY 12572
914-876-7082

TransPacific Health Products
3924 Central Avenue
St. Petersburg, FL 33711
800-336-9636
Chinese herbal formulas.

Homeopathy Organizations

American Institute of Homeopathy (AIH)
801 N. Fairfax Street, Suite 306
Alexandria, VA 22314
703-273-5250

John Bastyr College of Naturopathic Medicine
14500 Juanita Drive NE
Bothell, WA 98011
206-823-1300

Hahnemann Medical Clinic
828 San Pablo Ave.
Albany, CA 94706
510-524-3117

International Foundation for Homeopathy (IFH)
P.O. Box 7
Edmonds, WA 98020
425-776-4147

National Center for Homeopathy (NCH)
801 N. Fairfax Street, Suite 306
Alexandria, VA 22314
703-548-7790

National College of Naturopathic Medicine
049 SW Porter Street
Portland OR 97201
503-499-4343

Directories of Homeopaths

Council for Homeopathic Certification 408-425-1423

National Center for Homeopathy 703-548-7790

There is also a great website for homeopathy
which has a directory of homeopaths listed by
state: http://www.dimensional.com/~stevew

Homeopathic Suppliers

Homeopathic remedies are available in a growing number of
health food stores and pharmacies. If you cannot locate a local
supplier for the remedies you need, the following companies
will send individual remedies to you by mail; many also supply
homeopathic remedy kits and books on homeopathy.

Boericke and Tafel, Inc.
2381 Circadian Way
Santa Rosa, CA 95407
800-876-9505

Boiron, USA
800-BLU-TUBE
800-264-7661 Consumer Information Line

Dolisos America, Inc.
3014 Rigel Ave.
Las Vegas, NV 89102
800-365-4767

Hahnemann Medical Clinic
828 San Pablo Ave.
Albany, CA 94706
510-524-3117

Homeopathic Educational Services
2124 Kittredge St.
Berkeley, CA 94704
510-649-0294; 800-359-9051

Acupuncture and Acupressure

American Academy of Medical Acupuncture
5820 Wilshire Boulevard, Suite 500
Los Angeles, CA 90036
213-937-5514; 213-937-0959 (fax)
KCKD71F@Prodigy.com
http://www.medicalacupuncture.org

American Association of Acupuncture and Oriental
Medicine
4101 Lake Boone Trail, Suite 201
Raleigh, NC 27607-6528
919-965-7546

American Association of Oriental Medicine
433 Front Street
Catasauqua, PA 18032
610-266-1433
    Call or write for a list of acupuncturists who meet their
standards.

National Commission for the Certification of Acupuncturists
1424 16th Ave. NW
Washington, DC 20036

Humor Therapy

The American Association of Therapeutic Humor
222 South Merrimac #303
St. Louis, MO 63105

Massage

American Massage Therapy Association
820 Davis St., Suite 1000
Evanston, IL 60201

Mind-Body Healing

Center for Mind-Body Medicine
5225 Connecticut Ave., NW, Suite 414
Washington, DC 20015
202-966-7338

Institute for the Study of Human Knowledge
P.O. Box 176
Los Altos, CA 94023
    Publishes a newsletter, *Mental Medicine Update*, edited
by David Sobel, M.D. and Robert Ornstein, Ph.D.

Yoga

Yoga Journal
2054 University Ave.
Berkeley, CA 94704

A comprehensive yoga resource, with articles and listings of classes and workshops nationally.

INDEX

ABOUT THE AUTHORS

STEVEN J. BOCK, M.D. and KENNETH BOCK, M.D., are board-certified Family Practice Physicians. In addition to traditional medical training, they have advanced training in natural medicine, allergies, herbal medicine, nutrition, homeopathy, acupuncture and stress management. In 1983, they together founded the Rhinebeck Health Center with the goal of providing the best of conventional medicine combined with the best of alternative therapies. They recently opened a second holistic health facility in Albany, New York, the Center for Progressive Medicine. Over the course of fifteen years, they have developed a program for treating asthma in children using this combined approach, which draws on their expertise in the treatment of allergies and immune system disorders. Dr. Steven Bock is the author of *Stay Young the Melatonin Way*. Dr. Kenneth Bock is the author of *The Road to Immunity*. Both doctors are clinical instructors in the Department of Family Medicine at Albany Medical College.

NANCY BRUNING has authored or coauthored twenty books, most of which integrate conventional and natural medicines. They include: *Natural Remedies for Colds and Flu; Ayurveda: The A–Z Guide to Healing Techniques from Ancient India; The MEND Clinic Guide to Natural Medicine for Menopause and Beyond; Healing Homeopathic Remedies; What You Can Do About Chronic Hair Loss; What You Can Do About Incontinence; Coping with Chemotherapy; The Real Vitamin and Mineral Book; The Natural*

Health Guide to Antioxidants: Using Vitamins and Other Supplements to Fight Disease, Boost Immunity, and Maintain Optimal Health; Breast Implants: Everything You Need to Know; and *Swimming for Total Fitness.*